Urinary Tract Infection

Abhay Rané • Ranan Dasgupta

Editors

Urinary Tract Infection

Clinical Perspectives on Urinary
Tract Infection

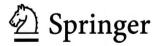 Springer

Editors
Abhay Rané, MS, FRCS, FRCS (Urol)
Department of Urology
Surrey and Sussex Healthcare NHS Trust
East Surrey Hospital
Redhill
UK

Ranan Dasgupta, MBBChir, MA, MD,
FRCS (Urol)
Department of Urology
Imperial College Healthcare NHS Trust
St Mary's Hospital
London
UK

ISBN 978-1-4471-4708-4   ISBN 978-1-4471-4709-1   (eBook)
DOI 10.1007/978-1-4471-4709-1
Springer London Heidelberg New York Dordrecht

Library of Congress Control Number: 2013942668

Printed on acid-free paper

Springer is part of Springer Science+Business Media (www.springer.com)

Foreword

Urinary tract infections (UTIs) constitute a significant health-care burden, affecting over 13 % of adult women yearly and comprising a lifetime prevalence of over 50 %. As such, the economic consequences and effect on quality of life of even routine UTIs are substantial. Add to that the impact of complicated UTIs – those infections occurring in patients with underlying anatomic abnormalities or those with urosepsis – and the effect on our health-care system is staggering.

The care of UTIs crosses medical disciplinary lines, falling to family practice doctors, obstetrician-gynecologists, internists, and urologists to diagnose and manage these problems. Thus, it behooves these clinicians to understand the underlying pathophysiology behind UTIs, to be able to differentiate simple from complicated UTIs, to be familiar with the diagnostic work-up, and finally to be comfortable with the treatment algorithm. Patients experiencing UTIs require acute diagnosis and management as well as potentially more detailed investigation and long-term care for those with recurrent UTIs. It is imperative that those patients at risk of or experiencing recurrent infections undergo appropriate evaluation to identify behavioral, genetic, or anatomic factors that contribute to their risk of UTIs.

In their book, *Urinary Tract Infection*, Abhay Rané and Ranan Dasgupta have assembled a group of well-known experts to author chapters addressing all aspects of UTI, including routine UTI; UTI complicated by diabetes, pregnancy, anatomic abnormalities, or indwelling catheters; UTI in children; and UTI associated with unusual organisms. Written in an easy-to-read question-answer format, this book addresses all aspects of clinical UTI, from pathogenesis to evaluation and treatment. Useful tables of antibiotic choices and dosages and signs and symptoms of UTI provide quick reference sources to which the busy practitioner can refer on the go. Applicable to practitioners in any specialty, this book provides a current, concise, yet comprehensive practical guide to the diagnosis and management of UTIs. I recommend this valuable publication be kept readily available on the shelf of any practitioner who cares for patients with UTIs.

Dallas, TX, USA   Margaret S. Pearle, MD, PhD

Preface

The causative organisms of urinary tract infection are dynamic in terms of their virulence and resistance patterns, leading to challenges in the prevention and treatment of urinary infection. This is of relevance in both primary and secondary care, and many of the challenges are similar in both developed and developing countries alike. UTI is also associated with considerable cost in terms of morbidity, economic, and research expenditure.

Written by an exceptional and well-known team of clinical experts, the purpose of *Clinical Perspectives on Urinary Tract Infections* is to address some key questions facing physicians about this condition. The book is written primarily for general physicians who wish to have a broad understanding of a number of important issues concerning infection in parts of the urinary tract. Specialists may also find the book useful as a quick reference guide.

We approach the subject from an organ-by-organ perspective, aware that patients may be affected systemically. By focusing on specific organs, it may help physicians to target investigation and management of underlying pathologies, as well as treating the infection by conventional antimicrobial measures.

Chapter 1 helps to define what is meant by "urinary tract infection" and describes the classification systems of common organisms. This leads on to Chap. 2, which discusses the main antibiotics used in treating these infections and includes discussion of antibiotic resistance, a growing problem on a global level.

Two very important areas of clinical dilemmas in UTI are comprehensively discussed next: pregnancy and children. These are followed by chapters on urinary tract infections and diabetes, less common infections, and a focus on UTI in AIDS and tuberculosis. Our final chapter discusses complementary therapies, such as plant-based supplements, nutritional formulas, and beverages.

In *Urinary Tract Infection*, we have utilized a question and answer style, which characterizes a clear and easy approach to learning and understanding, and which readers have found stimulating and helpful for information retention. The attractive handbook format makes the publication simple to carry and access and provides quick reference to those points that are of most interest. We hope you find the book informative and useful to your needs.

Redhill, UK   Abhay Rané, MS, FRCS, FRCS (Urol)

Acknowledgments

We wish to thank the team of extremely talented authors that have helped us put this book together. We also formally wish to acknowledge the support from Melissa Morton at Springer, and the dedication and hard work put in by our developmental editor, Portia Wong.

Finally, such an effort would not be complete without acknowledging our better halves: for their patience, understanding and words of encouragement, Ruta and Nina, we thank you.

Abhay Rané, MS, FRCS, FRCS (Urol)
Ranan Dasgupta, MBBChir, MA, MD, FRCS (Urol)

Contents

Contributors

Editors

Ranan Dasgupta, MBBChir, MA, MD, FRCS (Urol) Department of Urology, Imperial College Healthcare NHS Trust, St Mary's Hospital, London, UK

Abhay Rané, MS, FRCS, FRCS (Urol) Department of Urology, Surrey and Sussex Healthcare NHS Trust, East Surrey Hospital, Redhill, UK

Authors

Christopher Chiu, MRCP, FRCPath, PhD Infectious Diseases and Microbiology, Centre for Respiratory Infection, National Heart and Lung Institute, London, UK

Daniel Cohen, BMedSc, MBChB, MRCS Department of Urology, Imperial College London, London, UK

Magnus Grabe, MD, PhD Department of Urology, Skåne University Hospital, Malmö, Sweden

Dominic King, BSc, MBChB, MEd, MRCS Division of Surgery, Department of Surgery and Cancer, Imperial College London, London, UK

Henry A. Lee, BSc, MBBCh, MRCS (Eng) Division of Surgery, Department of Surgery and Cancer, Imperial College London, London, UK

Uwais Bashir Mufti, MBBSc, MRCS Department of Urology and Molecular Oncology, Imperial Healthcare NHS Trust, Charing Cross Hospital, London, UK

Taufiq Shaikh Charing Cross Hospital, Imperial College Healthcare NHS Trust, London, UK

Andrew Symes, MBBS, BSc, MD, FRCS (Urol) Department of Urology, Brighton and Sussex University Hospitals NHS Trust, Brighton, UK

Chapter 1
Definitions, Classifications, and Antibiotics

Christopher Chiu

Abstract Urinary tract infections (UTIs) are among the most common of all bacterial infections. They are an important cause of morbidity and mortality with a spectrum of severity that ranges from mild self-limiting infection to life-threatening systemic disease. Although they are commonly curable with antibiotics, widespread use of antimicrobials has inevitably led to a massive increase in UTIs caused by drug-resistant organisms. This has made antibiotic choice for empirical and rational treatment increasingly difficult. Here, we discuss the microbiology of UTIs, including the organisms that cause them, the interplay between bacteria and host that causes disease, mechanisms of antibiotic resistance, and factors influencing the choice of antibiotic for treatment. Through further understanding of the biology of the bacterial pathogens that cause UTIs, we aim to promote more responsible antibiotic prescribing in order to slow the pandemic spread of multiresistant organisms.

Keywords Bacteria • Antibiotics • Resistance • Pathogenesis • Risk factors • ESBL • AmpC • VRE

Definitions, Classifications, and Antibiotics

Urinary tract infection (UTI) may be defined as the presence of pathogens in the urinary tract. They are among the most common of bacterial infections and are frequent causes of morbidity and mortality. As the second most common reason for the prescription of empirical antibiotics, UTIs are also major drivers of antibiotic usage and antibiotic resistance. It is therefore essential that we understand the

C. Chiu, MRCP, FRCPath, PhD
Infectious Diseases and Microbiology, Centre for Respiratory Infection,
National Heart and Lung Institute, London, UK
e-mail: c.chiu@imperial.ac.uk

A. Rané, R. Dasgupta (eds.), *Urinary Tract Infection*,
DOI 10.1007/978-1-4471-4709-1_1, © Springer-Verlag London 2013

Table 1.1 Common definitions

Bacteriuria	Bacteria in urine, as demonstrated by microscopy or quantitative culture
Pyuria	$\geq 10^4$ white blood cells per milliliter of urine
Hematuria	Blood in the urine, either visible to the naked eye (macroscopic) or invisible to the naked eye (microscopic)
Significant bacteriuria	$\geq 10^4$ colony-forming units/ml of bacteria (usually of a single species) in a fresh urine specimen
Symptomatic bacteriuria	Bacteria in urine in the context of typical symptoms of UTI
Asymptomatic bacteriuria	Bacteria in urine in the absence of symptoms of UTI on at least two consecutive occasions
Urosepsis	UTI with accompanying sepsis syndrome

pathogenesis of these conditions so that they can be managed appropriately, not only for the benefit of the individual patient but also in order to control the spread of multidrug-resistant organisms.

How Common Are Urinary Tract Infections?

UTIs are extremely common, accounting for an estimated seven to ten million adult physician office visits each year in the USA [1] and 1–3 % of consultations in the UK general practice [2]. They are most frequent in infants, young women, and the elderly, with around a third of women by the age of 24 years having suffered a UTI requiring treatment and around 50 % of women having had an episode of UTI in their lifetime. Overall, UTIs are around twice as common in women as in men.

Invasive infections of the urinary tract, such as pyelonephritis, are less common, with around 250,000 cases per annum in the USA leading to around 200,000 admissions (1997 National Inpatient Sample database).

How Are Urinary Tract Infections Defined?

The mainstay of diagnosis of UTIs remains microscopy and culture of urine samples. The words used to describe UTIs are therefore generally couched in those terms (Table 1.1).

How May Urinary Tract Infections Be Classified and How Do These Assist in Clinical Management?

UTIs are generally classified according to their anatomical location or in terms of their severity and/or complexity.

Lower UTI, a term which encompasses *cystitis* and *urethritis*, is generally a benign condition that causes the typical symptoms of dysuria, suprapubic pain, frequency of micturition, urgency, hesitancy, and incomplete voiding. Systemic manifestations, such as fever, are uncommon and long-term sequelae are rare. It is usually treated with oral antibiotics which are excreted by the kidneys, thus reaching high levels in the urine, but not necessarily achieving high systemic or tissue levels.

Upper UTI or *pyelonephritis* is an invasive infection of the renal parenchyma, classically presenting with the triad of fever, renal angle tenderness, and nausea and vomiting. Lower urinary tract symptoms may or may not be present. Upper tract infections frequently cause *urosepsis*, and complications including kidney damage, abscess formation, and renal failure are common. Most cases will require admission and treatment with intravenous antibiotics that treat both the urinary and systemic components of the infection.

Uncomplicated UTIs are generally defined as lower tract infections affecting women with no structural, metabolic, or immunological predispositions. Some authorities also group cases of pyelonephritis with no complications in this category. Uncomplicated UTIs can be treated with narrower spectrum, oral antibiotics for short courses.

Complicated UTIs are those that involve the upper urinary tract and/or occur in individuals with predisposing factors such as structural and functional abnormalities, metabolic disorders, or impaired immunity. UTIs in children and men are often considered within this group, as UTI in these individuals is more frequently associated with predisposing factors, including congenital abnormalities in children and prostatitis in men. Many cases will require more protracted courses of broader spectrum antibiotics as multiresistant organisms are more common causes of these infections.

Recurrent UTIs: many women suffer recurrent infections. Recurrences may be divided into "relapses" where symptoms recur on cessation of treatment and the same organism is isolated or "reinfection" where a new causative organism is isolated. These patients are often exposed to multiple course of antibiotics or long-term antibiotic prophylaxis and may therefore rapidly develop infections with multiresistant organisms that render antibiotic choice problematic. In these cases, it may be important to explore non-pharmacological methods to reduce recurrences, such as improved hygiene and cranberry juice.

Why Do Urinary Tract Infections Occur?

There are two major routes by which microbial pathogens can infect the urinary tract: ascending spread of fecal flora and hematogenous spread. In addition to this, a variety of host factors affecting urine flow and local immunity predispose to colonization and infection by bacteria.

By far the most common route of infection is migration of organisms from the perineum via the urethra to the bladder and then to the kidney. Around 95 % of UTIs are thought to arise in this way. This explains the much greater incidence in young sexually active women in whom uropathogenic bacteria from the fecal flora are

Table 1.2 Types of bacteria causing urinary tract infection

	% Uncomplicated	% Complicated
Gram negative		
Escherichia coli	70–95	21–54
Proteus mirabilis	1–2	1–10
Klebsiella spp.	1–2	2–17
Citrobacter spp.	<1	5
Enterobacter spp.	<1	2–10
Pseudomonas aeruginosa	<1	2–19
Others	<1	6–20
Gram positive		
Staphylococcus saprophyticus	5–10	1–4
Enterococcus spp.	1–2	1–23
Group B streptococcus	<1	1–4
Staphylococcus aureus	<1	1–23
Others	<1	2

Adapted from. [9]

physically translocated via the short female urethra to infect the normally sterile urinary tract.

Only around 5 % of cases are due to infection following bacteremia. A number of pathogens, such as *Mycobacterium tuberculosis*, can spread to the renal tract in this way, although these are uncommon in the developed world.

Which Organisms Cause Urinary Tract Infections?

The majority of bacteria causing UTIs originate from the bowel, with a small percentage arising from skin flora (Table 1.2). Most data regarding mechanisms of pathogenicity have been obtained by study of *E. coli* which is the most common cause of both uncomplicated and complicated UTI. Bacteria express a variety of surface proteins, known as adhesins, which allow them to cling to epithelial cells. Uropathogenic *E. coli* may, for example, express P fimbriae which attach to globoseries-type glycolipids on urinary epithelium. These are found more commonly in strains that cause urosepsis. Other virulence factors, such as capsular polysaccharides, may protect against host defenses such as opsonization and phagocytosis, while a number of toxins, including alpha hemolysin and cytotoxic necrotizing factor 1, may be involved in local cellular damage.

Why Are Some Individuals More at Risk of Urinary Tract Infections?

UTIs occur when bacteria enter the urinary tract. If this happens more frequently or a greater bacterial load is introduced, for example, in sexually active women, poor hygiene, or instrumentation, the incidence of UTI increases. Furthermore, while host defenses (both physical and immunological) often destroy these pathogens before they establish an infection, impairment of these mechanisms will also predispose to infection. Predisposing factors include:

1. Structural and functional abnormalities: disruption of the normal flow of urine leads to urinary stasis. Under these conditions, bacteria can grow and divide more easily, leading to a greater bacterial load and increased likelihood of epithelial adhesion. These include congenital abnormalities, cysts and diverticula, and neurological defects causing urinary retention.
2. Foreign bodies: calculi and urinary catheters not only cause urinary turbulence but also act as nidus of infection where organisms settle and form biofilms. When bacteria, such as *Klebsiella* spp., start growing on solid matrices, they upregulate genes which promote the secretion of extracellular proteins as well as altering their metabolism in order to form a mucoid biofilm which is protective against the host immune response and prevents the penetration of antibiotics. Where a biofilm has formed on a foreign body, antibiotic therapy may be ineffective or only partially effective, promoting an environment that encourages resistance mutations to be selected. Some organisms, such as *Proteus* spp., produce urease enzymes that split urea, raising the pH of the urine and predisposing to the formation of calculi.
3. Metabolic abnormalities: glycosuria in diabetes mellitus and pregnancy encourages the growth of bacteria. Changes to the urinary epithelium also occur during pregnancy which may predispose to infection. Metabolic abnormalities may also lead to calculus formation.
4. Impaired immunity: increasing use of immunosuppressive drugs and solid organ and bone marrow transplantation have increased the risk of UTI and urosepsis in these patients. Although AIDS is now less common in the developed world due to the widespread use of antiretroviral therapy, immunosuppression due to HIV will also predispose to infections of the urinary tract.

Which Antibiotics Are Used for Empirical Treatment of Urinary Tract Infections?

Empirical antibiotics are those chosen when the exact causative organism and resistance pattern is unknown. In the case of UTI, the choice of antibiotics depends on a number of factors, including the relative prevalence of uropathogenic organisms, the local resistance patterns and levels of resistance previously observed, the clinical syndrome with which the patient presents and the origin of the infection, whether community-acquired or nosocomial. An empirical antibiotic for the treatment of UTIs should therefore have activity against the Gram-negative Enterobacteriaceae (such as *E. coli* and *Klebsiella* spp.) and Gram-positive organisms including *Staphylococcus saprophyticus* and ideally *Enterococcus* spp.

Uncomplicated, lower UTIs can be treated with oral antibiotics and should be restricted to short courses of 3–5 days if possible. Antibiotics such as nitrofurantoin, trimethoprim, and first-generation cephalosporins such as cephalexin are concentrated in the urine and therefore reach high levels above the minimum inhibitory concentrations (MIC) of most community-acquired organisms. The proportion of organisms found to be resistant to amoxicillin in most areas is now too high for this to be used as empirical therapy, although it is still the drug of choice for the treatment of most infections with *Enterococcus faecalis*. In some areas, resistance to trimethoprim, nitrofurantoin, and cephalexin is approaching levels where their use as empirical antibiotics may no longer be desirable, and alternative choices, such as quinolones, may be required.

Complicated UTIs require therapy with antibiotics that reach high systemic levels in order to treat bacteremia and invasive tissue infections such as pyelonephritis. Commonly used antibiotics include second-generation cephalosporins such as cefuroxime, co-amoxiclav, or ciprofloxacin. These may be supplemented with an aminoglycoside, such as gentamicin, which confers the benefit of rapid bactericidal activity as well as the addition of a second antibiotic class, thus increasing the likelihood of having treated early with an effective empirical antibiotic.

The exact choice of empirical antibiotics is highly dependent on the likelihood of resistant mutants within both the community and the individual patient. It is therefore important to take a full clinical history, as certain patient groups may require early treatment with broad-spectrum antibiotics. In particular, patients who have had recent inpatient admissions, recurrent courses of antibiotics, or reside in nursing homes are all at greater risk of infection with multiresistant organisms, including extended-spectrum beta-lactamase (ESBL) and AmpC producers (see below).

Why Is Bacterial Culture and Sensitivity Testing Important?

Empirical antibiotics are chosen on the basis of being sufficiently broad spectrum to treat the majority of UTIs in a patient group but sufficiently narrow spectrum to minimize attendant adverse effects, such as *Clostridium difficile*-associated diarrhea. However, for a proportion of cases, the first-line antibiotic choice will either be excessively broad (in the case of infection with very sensitive organisms) or have insufficient activity (where infecting organisms have intrinsic or acquired resistance). In both situations, it is desirable to have identified the causative organism and its sensitivity pattern so that antibiotic therapy can be rationalized appropriately.

How Has Antibiotic Resistance Arisen in Bacteria?

Many bacteria are intrinsically resistant to certain classes of antibiotics. These are due to characteristics encoded on the bacterial chromosome and include structural features, such as the outer membrane of most Gram-negative organisms which prevents penetration of vancomycin; the absence of antibiotic targets, such as the absence of cell wall in *Chlamydia* spp.; and membrane proteins such as efflux pumps that actively exclude antibiotics from the bacterial cell. Intrinsic resistance mechanisms are common to all members of a bacterial species and are not easily transferred to other species. They are therefore perceived as a lesser infection control risk.

The widespread use of antibiotics in medicine and agriculture has led to massive selection pressure on bacteria in our environment. Many organisms have acquired resistance mechanisms by either mutation or transfer of resistance genes via transposable genetic elements, including transposons and plasmids, which can spread rapidly within bacterial cells and between bacterial species. Many resistance genes are transferred together on the same plasmid and can therefore lead to the acquisition of multiple resistance phenotypes in a single step.

The most prevalent acquired resistance mechanisms are:

1. Alteration of the antibiotic target site:

    (a) Resistance to quinolones is commonly due to point mutations in DNA gyrase.
    (b) Resistance to tetracyclines occurs by mutations in dihydrofolate reductase.
    (c) The MecA gene in MRSA codes for a penicillin-binding protein that is not affected by methicillin/flucloxacillin.
    (d) The VanA gene cluster in vancomycin-resistant Enterococci (VRE) alters one of the components of the cell wall, preventing the binding of glycopeptides.

2. Alteration of the antibiotic

    (a) Beta-lactamases digest beta-lactam antibiotics with varying degrees of effectiveness, from simple penicillinases to extended-spectrum beta-lactamases (ESBLs) that can destroy all penicillins and most cephalosporins.
    (b) Acetyltransferases, adenytransferases, and phosphotransferases modify aminoglycosides, thus inhibiting their activity.

3. Efflux pumps

What Are Extended-Spectrum Beta-Lactamases (ESBLs)?

A number of Gram-negative bacteria possess intrinsic beta-lactam resistance mediated by chromosomal beta-lactamase genes which probably evolved in response to organisms such as beta-lactam-producing fungi [3]. However, the rapid spread of beta-lactamases is primarily due to the appearance of plasmid-mediated beta-lactamase genes, the first of which was discovered in the 1960s in *E. coli* and named TEM-1 [4]. Other beta-lactamases such as SHV-1, which is chromosomal in *Klebsiella pneumoniae* but generally plasmid-encoded in *E. coli*, have also become increasingly common.

Table 1.3 Bacteria with chromosomally encoded, inducible AmpC beta-lactamase

Enterobacter spp.
Serratia spp.
Citrobacter spp.
Acinetobacter spp.
Providencia spp.
Pseudomonas spp.
Morganella spp.

As these resistant organisms became a clinical problem, newer classes of antibiotics were developed with the specific intention of overcoming their resistance mechanisms. However, the pressure that these novel antibiotics exerted quickly led to the selection of mutants with beta-lactamase variants which were now able to hydrolyze them. In the mid-1980s, the first ESBL (SHV-2) was identified in a strain of *Klebsiella ozaenae* [5]. Functionally, organisms possessing these enzymes are resistant to third-generation cephalosporins but are inhibited by clavulanate which allows them to be identified on phenotypic testing.

The presence of ESBL genes on mobile genetic elements has allowed their rapid spread and also led to wide geographical variability in their incidence. While up to 40 % of *K. pneumoniae* isolates in France are resistant to ceftazidime [6], less than 1 % of *E. coli* and *K. pneumoniae* in the Netherlands are ESBL-producers [7]. In the United Kingdom during the 1990s, reports of resistant Gram-negative organisms with the ESBL phenotype were mainly derived from cases of nosocomial infection, primarily from intensive care units. These were caused by organisms carrying TEM or SHV genes and although intermittent outbreaks did occur these were not considered a widespread clinical problem [8].

In 2000, the first CTX-M gene was identified in the UK from an isolate of *K. oxytoca* and was rapidly followed by the emergence of ESBLs as a significant public health issue. By 2003, many laboratories in the UK were reporting organisms possessing CTX-M genes isolated from community patients, which differed markedly from the preceding trend in ESBLs. These organisms frequently also possessed other resistance mechanisms protecting them from the effects of quinolones and aminoglycosides.

What Are AmpC Beta-Lactamases and Which Organisms Produce Them?

ESBLs of the CTX-M group show significant structural similarity to AmpC beta-lactamases which are encoded on the chromosomes of several species of Enterobacteriaceae (Table 1.3).

In the majority of these, the AmpC gene is under the control of an inducible promoter and is therefore only produced at high levels when stimulated by the presence of antibiotics locally. More recently, mutations in the promoter have led to strains producing constitutively high levels of AmpC beta-lactamase. These genes have also increasingly transferred to plasmids which have spread to *E. coli* and *Klebsiella* spp., where again the protein is expressed at high levels, conferring resistance to all penicillins and first-, second-, and third-generation cephalosporins.

Which Antibiotics May Be Effective Against ESBL and AmpC Producers?

Carbapenems, including meropenem, imipenem, and ertapenem, are generally considered the treatment of choice for multiresistant Enterobacteriaceae. Although ESBLs are blocked by beta-lactamase inhibitors such as clavulanic acid and tazobactam, antibiotic combinations containing these are unreliable in vivo. These organisms are sometimes sensitive to quinolones and aminoglycosides, in which case they may be used to spare carbapenem use, but often there are few choices of antibiotics available against very resistant isolates.

The increasing use of carbapenems has inevitably encouraged the appearance of carbapenemase-producing organisms. In order to reduce the reliance on this drug class and the resulting selection pressure, newer antibiotics have been developed such as tigecycline, and older drugs have been resurrected (e.g., temocillin) which are resistant to hydrolysis by ESBLs and AmpCs, although resistance against these antibiotics also exists. In the case of multiresistant *Pseudomonas* spp. or *Acinetobacter baumannii*, which can carry multiple resistance mechanisms and has caused severe nosocomial outbreaks, it may be necessary to treat with more toxic drugs such as colistin.

What Are Vancomycin-Resistant Enterococci (VRE)?

Use of cephalosporins selects for enterococci which are part of the normal bowel flora and are intrinsically resistant to cephalosporins. They have therefore become more common as causes of UTI. Furthermore, increased nosocomial use of vancomycin for the treatment of MRSA and *C. difficile*-associated diarrhea has encouraged the spread of VREs which are commonly resistant to all glycopeptides with variable sensitivity to aminopenicillins, depending on the species. Although often found colonizing non-sterile sites rather than truly causing infections, antibiotic choice is limited when treating VREs.

What Antibiotics May Be Effective Against VRE?

If the isolate is sensitive, amoxicillin is the treatment of choice for VRE. However, although the most commonly isolated species, *Enterococcus faecalis*, is usually sensitive to amoxicillin, most others are not. Conversely, *E. faecalis* is intrinsically resistant to quinupristin/dalfopristin (Synercid) while other species are sensitive.

Linezolid is now widely used for infections with amoxicillin-resistant VRE. Other newer antibiotics including tigecycline and daptomycin also have activity against most isolates.

Key Points
- Urinary tract infections are very common.
- They are most common in sexually active women, young children, and the elderly.
- UTIs are usually due to translocation of bacteria originating from the bowel ascending into the urinary tract.
- Lower, uncomplicated UTIs have no long-term sequelae and are generally treated with short courses of oral antibiotics.
- Pyelonephritis, urosepsis, and other complicated UTIs usually require hospital admission and intravenous antibiotics.
- Urine and blood culture with sensitivity testing is essential in order to rationalize the antibiotic choice.
- Widespread antibiotic use has promoted the spread of resistance.
- Among the Gram-negative Enterobacteriaceae, the prevalence of ESBL and AmpC-producing organisms is increasing in both hospital and community settings.
- Multiresistant organisms may require treatment with very broad-spectrum antibiotics and newer antibiotic classes.

References

1. Foxman B. Epidemiology of urinary tract infections: incidence, morbidity, and economic costs. Dis Mon. 2003;49:53–70.
2. Office of Population Censuses and Statistics. Morbidity statistics from general practice.Fourth national study 1991-92. London: OPCS, 1996.
3. Ghuysen JM. Serine beta-lactamases and penicillin-binding proteins. Annu Rev Microbiol. 1991;45:37–67.
4. Marchandin H, Carriere C, Sirot D, Pierre HJ, Darbas H. TEM-24 produced by four different species of Enterobacteriaceae, including Providencia rettgeri, in a single patient. Antimicrob Agents Chemother. 1999;43:2069–73.
5. Kliebe C, Nies BA, Meyer JF, Tolxdorff-Neutzling RM, Wiedemann B. Evolution of plasmid-coded resistance to broad-spectrum cephalosporins. Antimicrob Agents Chemother. 1985;28:302–7.
6. Branger C, Lesimple AL, Bruneau B, Berry P, Lambert-Zechovsky N. Long-term investigation of the clonal dissemination of Klebsiella pneumoniae isolates producing extended-spectrum beta-lactamases in a university hospital. J Med Microbiol. 1998;47:201–9.
7. Stobberingh EE, et al. Occurrence of extended-spectrum betalactamases (ESBL) in Dutch hospitals. Infection. 1999;27:348–54.
8. Livermore DM, Hawkey PM. CTX-M: changing the face of ESBLs in the UK. J Antimicrob Chemother. 2005;56:451–4.
9. Hooton TM. The current management strategies for community-acquired urinary tract infection. Infect Dis Clin North Am. 2003 Jun;17(2):303–32. Review.

Chapter 2
Diagnosis and Management of Infections of the Urinary Tract

Magnus Grabe

Abstract Urinary tract infections are among the most frequent infections encountered in both the community and the hospital environment. They range from harmless asymptomatic bacteriuria and self-curing cystitis to severe pyelonephritis with life-threatening sepsis. *Escherichia coli* is the most common gram-negative urinary tract pathogen followed by *Proteus* sp., *Klebsiella* sp., and other *Enterobacteriaceae*. Gram-positive species such as *Enterococci* and *Staphylococcus* spp. are often found in urine culture.

Early diagnoses and determination of the severity of the infection are necessary for an effective medical treatment. Urological patients are particularly prone to urinary tract infections, and the identification of a possible risk factor requiring a surgical intervention or drainage can be vital to the patient.

In view of the worsening resistance pattern of common urinary pathogens against available antibiotics, it is important to comply with evidence-based, recommended treatment regimens.

Keywords Asymptomatic bacteriuria • Cystitis • Pyelonephritis • Risk factors for urinary tract infections • Sepsis • Urine culture • Urinary tract infection

What Is an Infection of the Urinary Tract?

The normal urinary tract is sterile. Urinary tract infection (UTI) is defined as an inflammatory response of the urothelium to the invasion of microorganisms, usually bacteria, also called uropathogens. The invasion of bacteria, as shown by bacterial growth on the culture of urine, is defined as bacteriuria. Symptomatic UTI is the

M. Grabe, MD, PhD
Department of Urology, Skåne University Hospital, Malmö SE-205 02, Sweden
e-mail: magnus.grabe@skane.se

A. Rané, R. Dasgupta (eds.), *Urinary Tract Infection*,
DOI 10.1007/978-1-4471-4709-1_2, © Springer-Verlag London 2013

presence of both bacteriuria and typical symptoms, while asymptomatic bacteriuria (ABU) is the presence of bacteriuria in the absence of symptoms. ABU in conjunction with an indwelling catheter is often referred to as colonization of the urinary tract.

Is UTI a Major Health Problem?

Urinary tract infections are among the most frequent infections encountered in the community. Catheter-associated infections account for approximately 30–40 % of the healthcare-associated infections (HAI) and are an important source of severe urinary tract infections and septicemia. Prevalence studies have shown that up to 10 % of patients in urological wards have healthcare-associated complicated infections.

What Is the Classification of UTI?

For practical reasons, it is reasonable to classify UTI as:

- Bacteriuria or colonization (presence of microorganisms in urine)
- Uncomplicated UTI (uUTI)

    - Cystitis
    - Uncomplicated pyelonephritis

- Complicated UTI (cUTI)

    - Febrile, upper UTI
    - Complicated pyelonephritis

- Sepsis

   It is understood that there is no known or detected underlying abnormality or dysfunction of the urinary tract in uUTI, while in cUTI there is one or several such complicating factors (Tables 2.1 and 2.2).

   UTI can be sporadic, recurrent, or reinfection. Usually there should go more than 6 months between episodes of UTI to speak about sporadic or isolated infections, while recurrent UTI are defined as three or more infections per year. Reinfections mean the acquisition of a new infection, while relapse is the reappearance of the same bacterial strain originating from a focus in the urinary tract, i.e., the prostate, a bladder diverticulum, and a kidney stone.

How Frequent Is Bacteriuria in the Population?

The overall prevalence of bacteriuria in the population is estimated to 3.5 %. Bacteriuria is present in schoolgirls in 1–2 % and young women in 1–5 %. The

Table 2.1 Main factors associated with complicated UTI

Factors associated with complicated UTI	Examples
Congenital anatomic and functional abnormality	Pelvio-ureteral junction (PUJ) obstruction
	Vesicoureteral reflux
	Congenital neurological disorder (i.e., myelomeningocele)
Obstruction of the urinary tract	Kidney stone disease
	Bladder outlet obstruction
	Residual urine
	Ureteral tumor
	Extrinsic compression of the ureter
	Ureteral stricture
Neurological dysfunction	Spinal cord injury
	Multiple sclerosis
	Stroke
Concomitant medical disorders	Diabetes mellitus
	Disorder of the immune system

Table 2.2 Factors that might increase the susceptibility to UTI

Factors	Examples
Genetic and familiar factors	Host response capacity
	Nonsecretor status
	ABO blood-group antigens
Biological factors	Congenital abnormalities
	Urinary tract obstruction
	Prior history of UTI
	Medical concomitant diseases (Table 2.1)
	Dysfunction of the urinary tract
	Renal transplant
	Immunologic abnormalities (i.e., HIV)
Behavioral	Sexual intercourse
	Some contraceptive devices (i.e., diaphragms, condoms, spermicides)
Urological surgery and instrumentation	Catheters/stents/foreign materials
	Infections associated with an instrument or operation
Others	Estrogen deficiency in aging women
	Previous use of antibiotics
	Long hospital stay
	Reduced mental status

rate is increasing with age, and it is estimated that some 25 % of all women over the age of 65 years living at their home have bacteriuria, while this figure range from 25 to 50 % in women cared for in institutions for elderly persons. All patients with indwelling catheters or other long-term urinary tract stents have bacteriuria.

How Frequent Is Symptomatic UTI in the Population?

The cumulative incidence of UTI through the age of 6 years is approximately 1 % in girls and 0.1–0.2 % in boys. One third of all women will have reported a UTI before the age of 24 years, and the cumulative probability of UTI in women is about 50 % at 50 years of age. There is a 40–50 % risk of a new infection within a few months.

Do Men Have UTI?

UTI in men are uncommon until the age of 50 years, when increasing bladder outlet obstruction is developing and markedly changes the odds of having a UTI. On the other hand, adult men are prone to bacterial prostatitis, a urogenital infection involving both the prostatic gland and the lower urinary tract (NIH prostatitis type I and II).

Which Are the Most Frequent Factors Associated with a cUTI?

Which Pathogens Cause UTI?

It is essential to know the likely causative pathogens for an appropriate antimicrobial treatment. Most UTI are caused by the microorganisms listed in Table 2.3. *Escherichia coli* is the most frequently encountered microbe, present in as many as 75–80 % of the community-acquired uUTI and approximately 35–50 % of the UTI. Other main gram-negative bacterial species are *Klebsiella* and *Proteus* spp., *Pseudomonas* sp. and gram-positive strains such as *Enterococcus faecalis*, and some *Staphylococci* species, i.e., *Staphylococcus epidermidis*, *Staphylococcus aureus*, and *Staphylococcus saprophyticus*, the latter usually only in female UTI.

Are There Other Specific Infections of the Urinary Tract?

Bacillus tuberculosis is causing progressive destruction and scares of the urinary tract with retained calcifications. Tuberculosis is still a worldwide infectious disease of major importance and hits the urinary tract in at least some 5–10 % of the cases. Also the blood fluke *Schistosoma haematobium* (bilharzias, snail fever) is endemic in defined geographic areas, producing fibrotic lesions, strictures, and scares of the ureter and bladder as well as being a possible underlying cause of bladder cancer.

Table 2.3 Classification of UTI, most frequent causative pathogens, and treatment recommendation

Type of UTI	Bacteria	Antibiotics	Length of treatment	Remarks
uUTI (sporadic) Cystitis	*E. coli* (75–80 %) *Proteus* spp. (≤5 %) *Klebsiella* spp. (≤5%) *S. saprophyticus* (5–10 %) *Enterococcus* spp. (<5 %)	TMP (+/− SMZ) Pivmecillinam Nitrofurantoin Fosfomycin 2G cephalosporins	3–5 days	Avoid F-quinolones
uUTI (recurrent)	Ditto	Ditto+ F-quinolones	7–10 days	
uUTI (pyelo-nephritis)	*E. coli* (75–80 %) *Proteus* spp. (≤5%) *Klebsiella* spp. (≤5%) *Others*	3G cephalosporins F-quinolones TMP+SMZ	7–14 days	Parenchymal infection
UTI in pregnancy	Ditto	Ref. to national recommendations	7 days	Long-term prophylaxis
cUTI	*E. coli* (35–50 %) *Proteus, Klebsiella, other Enterobacteriacae* spp. (15–25 %) *Pseudomonas* (5–15 %) *Enterococcus* (5–20 %) *Others* (<10 %)	3G cephalosporins F-quinolones TMP+SMZ Aminoglycosides	10–14 days	Empirical treatment. adjustment according to culture result
Acute bacterial prostatitis (NIH type I)	*E. coli* Other uropathogens	3G cephalosporins F-quinolones TMP+SMZ Aminoglycosides	≥14 days	Consider *Chlamydia* infection in young men
Septicemia	*E. coli* (35–50 %) *Proteus, Klebsiella, other Enterobacteriacae* spp. (15–25 %) *Pseudomonas* (5–15 %) *Enterococcus* (5–20 %) *Others* (<10 %)	3G cephalosporins F-quinolones TMP+SMZ Aminoglycosides	10–14 days	2 AB General supportive treatment
Catheter-associated UTI	*E. coli* *Proteus, Klebsiella, Enterococcus faecalis* spp. *Pseudomonas* spp. *Others*	According to culture	5–10 days	No AB in ABU Only symptom-atic UTI

uUTI uncomplicated urinary tract infection, *cUTI* complicated urinary tract infection, *TMP* trimethoprim, *SMZ* sulfamethoxazole, *Spp* species, *2G and 3G* second and third generation, *AB* antibiotic, *ABU* asymptomatic bacteriuria

What Is the Pathogenesis of UTI?

The bowel constitutes the reservoir of the microorganisms colonizing the urogenital tracts. *E. coli* infections have been extensively studied and are caused by a disturbance in the host-parasite balance. The vagina, periurethral zone, and even the urethra are naturally colonized by microorganisms originating from the fecal flora and the perineal skin. *E. coli* adheres to the uro-epithelium through adhesines (P fimbriae and type 1 fimbriae). The bacteria can also express toxins such as α-hemolysin and cytotoxic necrotic factor 1.

The hosts' defense is relying on specific local and systemic antibodies and the inflammatory response. The bacterial adhesion to the epithelium produces a signal and activation of the cellular defense functions. Chemokines are released, stimulating a neutrophil recruitment. In UTI, the more severe the infection, the higher is the expression of virulence factors. In ABU, there is an attenuation of virulence factors, whereas in uncomplicated pyelonephritis, the expression is usually high. The more compromised the natural defense mechanisms of the host, the fewer the expression of virulence. There are indications that some individuals are genetically more susceptible to UTI.

Are There Any Risk Factors?

A wide range of factors have been identified that can increase susceptibility to UTI (Table 2.2). An intrinsic factor is a factor harbored within the patient such as a genetic, biological, or functional abnormality. An extrinsic factor is related to external features such as hygiene and behavior, the introduction of a catheter, and urological instrumentation.

What Are the Most Common Symptoms?

The most frequent symptoms and clinical signs of UTI are:

- Dysuria, urgency, frequency, and suprapubic tenderness for the lower urinary tract
- Fever and abdominal or flank pain, usually accompanied by flank tenderness, and nausea as signs of a febrile upper UTI or pyelonephritis
- Chills and shivering as signs of bacteremia
- Circulatory instability and eventually organ failure as signs of sepsis

How to Diagnose a UTI?

The diagnosis of a UTI is based on the combination of symptoms and laboratory findings.

Urine dipstick test for leukocytes esterase and nitrate is basic, easy, and reliable in most infections. The first demonstrate the presence of leukocytes in the urine or pyuria (≥ 10 WBC/mm^3). The second displays the presence of bacteria. Consistent pyuria with a series of negative urine culture leads to the suspicion of a specific infection.

Bacterial count in terms of *colony-forming units* (cfu) is important. For sporadic cystitis in women, a bacterial count of $\geq 10^3$ cfu/mL is accepted, while $\geq 10^4$ cfu/mL is necessary to define an uncomplicated pyelonephritis. A cUTI requires the same symptoms and $\geq 10^4$ cfu/mL in females and $\geq 10^5$ cfu/mL in males. ABU is defined as the presence of $\geq 10^5$ cfu/mL in at least two consecutive cultures in an otherwise symptom-free individual.

A midstream urine culture (MSU culture) is followed by a susceptibility testing that will guide in the choice of antibiotics.

Basic blood samples are collected for hemoglobin, white blood cells (WBC) and differential count, C-reactive protein (CRP), and S-creatinine. Sampling is unnecessary in sporadic uUTI but highly recommended in uncomplicated pyelonephritis and UTI as part of the diagnostic process.

In case of high fever, chills, and clinical suspicion of severe upper UTI and/or septicemia, it is essential to collect at least two samples of blood for blood culture. Imaging of the urinary tract is required in recurrent infections, in case of febrile infection or when a complicating factor is suspected. Radiological evaluation is also done in case of treatment failure. This can be done with an ultrasound examination, an intravenous pyelogram, or a computerized tomography, depending on the clinical situation and available methods.

What Are the Principles of Management of UTI?

There are three main aims in the management of UTI:

- Effective therapeutic response
- Prevention of recurrence
- Reduce the development of resistance of bacterial strains

How Do You Treat an Uncomplicated UTI?

Cystitis is the most common UTI, involving only the lower urinary tract, and is seen in both pre- and postmenopausal women. There is no fundamental difference in the principle of treatment. However, with increased age, the recurrence rate may increase and, thus, the regimens length.

In sporadic UTI, empiric treatment can be initiated on the basis of symptoms without any further workup. A short treatment of 3–5 days is sufficient (Table 2.3). No clinical or microbiological follow-up is usually required. However, if therapy fails, laboratory testing should be undertaken.

A more thorough diagnostic evaluation is indicated for women with evidence of uncomplicated pyelonephritis. This workup includes a urine analysis, urine culture and susceptibility testing, blood samples, and, when considered as necessary, radiological evaluation. Involving the renal parenchyma, this infection is more serious and requires a 7–14-day treatment. Clinical and microbiological follow-up is recommended.

How Do You Treat a Recurrent UTI?

Recurrent UTI is defined as three or more infections within a year. Recurrent UTI are seen in women with a family history of UTI and limited intake of fluids and few voiding occasions. Sexual intercourse and some contraceptive measures may increase the frequency of UTI. In elderly women, prolapse, intestinal troubles, and concomitant diseases such as diabetes are underlying causes for recurrent UTI. Patients with recurrent UTI should be investigated for any anatomical or functional abnormality by imaging of the urinary tract, cystoscopy, and urodynamic studies as required.

In men, recurrent bacteriuria and urogenital infections can be caused by a chronic bacterial prostatitis (NIH type II). Clinical and microbiological follow-up is recommended.

Are There Any Preventive Measures Against Recurrence?

There is little evidence for each of the different measures that are usually given as recommendation to women with recurrent UTI. It is essential to inform and promote an understanding of the reasons for recurrence and to detect any underlying cause.

General advice includes:

- A high intake of fluids
- Regular urination in order to avoid distension of the bladder and residual urine with bacterial growth opportunities
- Good hygiene and postcoital voiding
- Avoidance of spermicides

Antibiotic prophylaxis reduces the number of episodes but is controversial in view of the development of antibiotic resistance. Short courses à la demand is an alternative. Both *cranberry* extracts (Vaccinium macrocarpon) and vaccination with bacterial extracts are under investigation.

What Is Acute Bacterial Prostatitis?

Acute bacterial prostatitis is a serious, usually febrile infection creating an inflammation of the glandular tissue. The condition is accompanied by dysuria, perineal pain, bladder outlet voiding symptoms, and fever. Inflammatory parameters such as CRP and white blood count are increased. In adult men, the causative microorganisms are the usually uropathogens, although sexually transmitted infections also have to be considered. In younger men, *Chlamydia* infection must be taken into account.

As for UTI, the treatment is empirical and initiated with an antibiotic covering the usual uropathogens until culture is available. It should last for at least 14 days. Clinical and microbiological follow-up is recommended.

What Is Different About a UTI During Pregnancy?

The consequences of UTI or untreated ABU during pregnancy can be significant, including an elevated risk of pyelonephritis, premature delivery, fetal mortality, and pregnancy-induced hypertension. Therefore, screening for bacteriuria is highly recommended. Owing to the seriousness of inadequate management during pregnancy, all infections should be adequately treated, usually for a period of 7–10 days, depending on the severity. Additionally, it is generally recommended to give long-term prophylaxis in case of ABU.

Should Asymptomatic Bacteriuria Be Treated?

It is recommended not to treat ABU except during pregnancy. Only episodes of symptomatic bacteriuria should be given antibiotics. The same recommendations as for UTI are valid. ABU must be controlled prior to urological surgery.

Should Catheter-Associated Infections Be Treated?

Asymptomatic infections associated with an indwelling catheter, a ureteral catheter or stent, or a nephrostomy tube should not be treated unless there are obvious signs of clinical infection. Only clinical significant infections are given antimicrobial agents.

How Do You Treat a Complicated UTI?

In case of high fever and/or shivering, a urine culture and two blood cultures are highly recommended. When a UTI is suspected, imaging investigation of the urinary tract for underlying cause and risk factor assessment is required. The treatment is combined:

- Medical with one or two antimicrobial agents
- Surgical, i.e., when drainage or other surgical measures are required

The medical treatment is empirical and initiated with at least one intravenous antibiotic for 1–3 days until the fever is controlled and the laboratory findings show a stabilization or decrease of the inflammatory process (Table 2.3). At the same time, the result of the urine culture and susceptibility of the microorganisms will be available, guiding in the choice of subsequent agents. It is important to note that former urine cultures can guide in the choice of the first antibiotics. Monitoring and full life-supportive measures have to be taken as requested. A clinical and microbiological follow-up is recommended.

What Is the Best Way to Treat a Sepsis?

Sepsis is a serious life-threatening condition requiring rigorous antibiotic treatment similar to that of UTI. Urine and blood cultures are imperative. Monitoring and full life-support treatment in cooperation with intensive care specialists is mandatory. Initial treatment with two antibiotics is recommended (Table 2.3). As for UTI, the treatment is both medical and surgical. Necessary imaging and potential causative factors, i.e., obstructive kidney stone, residual urine, and tumor disease, have to be detected early and managed properly. The same follow-up as for UTI is recommended.

Which Antibiotic(s) Should Be Used to Treat UTI?

The most useful antibiotics for the different types of infections are listed in Table 2.4. Uncomplicated UTI are treated with short 3- to 5-day courses with trimethoprim, trimethoprim-sulfamethoxazole, nitrofurantoin, pivmecillinam, or fosfomycin, when available. It is essential to avoid fluoroquinolones for lower UTI.

Uncomplicated pyelonephritis can usually be treated for 7–14 days with trimethoprim-sulfamethoxazole or a fluoroquinolone. β-lactam penicillins with a β-lactamase inhibitor, cephalosporins, fluoroquinolones, and aminoglycosides are useful for UTI and sepsis.

In pregnancy, β-lactam antibiotics and nitrofurantoin can be given, while fluoroquinolones, tetracyclines, and even trimethoprim are to be avoided due to the risk of adverse effects on fetal development.

What Are the Main Risks with Antibiotics?

All antibiotics can induce hypersensitive reactions of immediate or delayed type; gastrointestinal side effects such as diarrhea, nausea, and vomiting; and hematological disorders, i.e., leucopoenia and thrombocytopenia. National pharmacopeia will give detailed adverse reactions, important interactions, and contraindications.

Table 2.4 List of the most common antimicrobial agents used for the treatment of uUTI and cUTI. The list below is indicative and mentions the most common side effects, interactions, and contraindication

Name	Mode of action	Dose (adults)	Main adverse effects (*see comments)	Important interactions and contraindications
Trimethoprim	Acid folic metabolism	160 mg ×2	GI disturbances Allergic reactions (skin rash)	Known hypersensitivity to trimethoprim Renal insufficiency Might interact with some contraceptive drugs, cyclosporine, and glibenclamide Avoid during first term of pregnancy
Trimethoprim + sulfamethoxazole	Acid folic metabolism	160/800 mg ×2 Reduce dose according to renal function	GI disturbances Allergic reactions (skin rash) Renal function reduction	Known hypersensitivity to trimethoprim and/or sulfamethoxazole Renal insufficiency Might interact with some contraceptive drugs, cyclosporine, and glibenclamide Avoid during pregnancy
Mecillinam Pivmecillinam	Bacterial cell wall synthesis	200 mg ×3 or 400 mg ×2	GI disturbances Allergic reaction (immediate or delayed)	Known hypersensitivity to beta-lactam antibiotics Interaction with probenecid Avoid during last month of pregnancy
Ampicillin + BLI	Bacterial cell wall synthesis	500–750 mg ×2	Dito mecillinam	Dito mecillinam
Cephalosporins	Bacterial cell wall synthesis	Depend on compound	GI disturbances	Risk for cross allergic reaction in known hypersensitivity to other beta-lactam antibiotics
Examples				
Cefotaxime (IV)		Dose adapted to clinical severity 1 g ×3 (IV)	Allergic reactions (immediate and delayed)	Interaction with probenecid
Cefadroxil (oral)		500 mg–1 g ×2		

(continued)

Table 2.4 (continued)

Name	Mode of action	Dose (adults)	Main adverse effects (*see comments)	Important interactions and contraindications
Nitrofurantoin	30S inhibitor	50 mg × 3	GI disturbances	Known glucose-6-phosphodehydrogenas deficiency
			Fever, headache, muscular pain Pulmonary lesion Leucopenia, anemia	Directly prior to delivery
Fosfomycin	Bacterial cell wall synthesis	3 g single dose	GI disturbances	Metoclopramide
F-quinolones (ciprofloxacin)	DNA gyrase/topoisomerase	Ciprofloxacin 250–500 mg × 2	GI disturbances	Hypersensitivity to F-quinolones
		Ofloxacin 200–400 mg × 2	Allergic reactions	Interaction with tizanidine, antacidum, dairy products, warfarin, etc.
		Dose adapted to clinical severity	Headache	History of quinolone-associated tendinitis
		Avoid in simple infections	Secondary infections	Dose reduction related to renal function
				Only on strict indication during pregnancy
Aminoglycosides	30S inhibitors	3–5 mg/kg/day divided in 3 equal doses.	Nephrotoxicity	Reduced renal function
Gentamicin		Tobramycin can be given in one initial dose in severe infection	Ototoxicity	Therapeutic levels control at 2–3 days or according to kidney function
Tobramycin			Vestibular toxicity	During pregnancy: only in very severe infections

For details on adverse effects and interactions, it is necessary to consult national pharmacological and treatment manuals and pharmacopeia of reference

All antibiotics can induce a secondary infection. The most common are gastro-intestinal infection with *Clostridium difficile*, particularly with cephalosporins, F-quinolones, and fungal infection (i.e., *Candida albicans* infection).

Is There a Threat with the Use of Antibiotics?

There is a growing worldwide threat in the development of multiresistant bacteria. This threat is to be taken seriously as at the end, even simple uncomplicated infection might become difficult to treat. There is a correlation between the use of antimicrobial agents and the development of resistant bacterial strains. The systematic use of some antibiotics produces also a collateral damage, selecting resistant strains in the community and the hospital environment. It is therefore recommended to reduce the prescription to the recommended regimens and to follow local and international guidelines in the management of UTI, as for other infections.

Key Points
- UTI are among the most frequent uncomplicated infections in the community. Indwelling catheters are the underlying cause of most of the healthcare-associated UTI, usually complicated and often severe.
- Urine culture is a key diagnostic tool. The result is obtained after that empiric treatment is initiated and leads to relevant adjustment according to the needs.
- Sporadic cystitis requires only a short 2- to 5-day treatment, while an ascending pyelonephritis needs a 7–14-day antibiotic treatment.
- Severe complicated UTI and Sepsis can be life-threatening. Treatment has to be initiated without any delay after primary clinical diagnosis.
- All antibiotics can give both gastrointestinal disturbances and allergic reactions. Knowledge about the renal function is important. Initial treatment can usually be started with normal dosage, but further doses must be adjusted to the renal function and the patient's general condition.
- Misuse of antibiotics leads inevitably to bacterial resistance development.

Further Reading

Bichler K-H, Savatovsky I, Naber KG, Bishop MC, et al. EAU guidelines for the management of urogenital schistosomiasis. Eur Urol. 2006;49:998–1003.

Bjerklund-Johansen T, Cek M, Naber K, Stratchounski L, et al. Prevalence of hospital-acquired urinary tract infections in Urology Departments. Eur Urol. 2007;51:1100–12.

Cek M, Lenk S, Naber KG, Bishop MC, et al. EAU guidelines for the management of genitourinary tuberculosis. Eur Urol. 2005;48:353–62.

Foxman B. Epidemiology of urinary tract infections: incidence, morbidity and economic costs. Am J Med. 2002;113:5S–13.

Grabe M, Bishop MC, Bjerklund Johansen TE, Botto H, et al. Urological infections. Guidelines of the European Association of Urology. Arnhem: EAU Guidelines Office. ISBN-13:978-90-79754-09-0. www.uroweb.com/professional-resources/guidelines/online/.

Marcel J-P, Alfa M, Banquero F, Etienne J, Goossens H, et al. Healthcare-associated infections: think globally, act locally. Clin Microbiol Infect. 2008;14:895–907.

Naber K, Schito G, Botto H, Palou J, Mazzei T. Surveillance Study in Europe and Brazil on clinical aspects and antimicrobial resistance epidemiology in females with cystitis (ARESC): implications for empiric therapy. Eur Urol. 2008;54:1164–78.

Nicolle LE. Urinary tract infection: traditional pharmacologic therapies. Am J Med. 2002; 113(1A):35S–44.

Ronald A. The etiology and urinary tract infection: traditional and emerging pathogens. Am J Med. 2002;113:14S–9.

Stamm WE. Scientific and clinical challenges in the management of urinary tract infections. Am J Med. 2002;113(1A):1S–4.

Svanborg C, Bergsten G, Fischer H, Godaly G, et al. Uropathogenic Escherichia coli as a model of host-parasite interaction. Curr Opin Microbiol. 2006;9:33–9. Available at: www.sciencedirect.com.

Tenke P, Kovacs B, Bjerklund Johansen T, Matsumoto T, et al. European and Asian guidelines on management and prevention of catheter-associated urinary tract infections. Int J Antimicrob Agents. 2008;31S:S68–78.

Wagenlehner F, Naber K. Treatment of bacterial urinary tract infections: presence and future. Eur Urol. 2006;49:235–44.

Chapter 3
Clinical Dilemmas

Daniel Cohen and Ranan Dasgupta

Abstract Pregnancy poses its own specific problems with regard to urinary infections, in terms of both treatment and prophylaxis. Certain antibiotics are safe in certain trimesters, and there is also evidence for the use of antibiotics in the management of asymptomatic bacteriuria during pregnancy, particularly to reduce the frequency of pyelonephritis and its sequelae.

Similarly the treatment of UTIs in childhood presents different challenges, particularly as the sequelae of this can present later in adulthood, and there are conditions such as phimosis and vesicoureteric reflux, the timing of the treatment of which can lead to controversies in management. Specialist care is recommended in these cases, and close follow-up through adolescence into adulthood would be beneficial.

Keywords Pregnancy • Bacteriuria • Antibiotics

Part I: UTI in Pregnancy

How Common Are UTIs During Pregnancy?

UTIs are the most common bacterial infections in pregnancy. Asymptomatic bacteriuria complicates between 4 and 10 % of all pregnancies. Up to 4 % of women will develop an acute cystitis during pregnancy, and 1–2 % will develop acute

D. Cohen, BMedSc, MBChB, MRCS
Department of Urology, Imperial College London, London, UK

R. Dasgupta, MBBChir, MA, MD, FRCS (Urol) (✉)
Department of Urology, Imperial College Healthcare NHS Trust,
St Mary's Hospital, Praed Street, London W2 1NY, UK
e-mail: ranandg@yahoo.co.uk

A. Rané, R. Dasgupta (eds.), *Urinary Tract Infection*,
DOI 10.1007/978-1-4471-4709-1_3, © Springer-Verlag London 2013

pyelonephritis, most commonly in the third trimester. This incidence is significantly higher than in the nonpregnant population.

Women with a previous history of UTIs, urinary tract abnormalities, and diabetes have an increased risk. There is also some evidence that women of lower socioeconomic class have higher rates of infection. There is a consensus view that pregnant women should be screened for bacteriuria at least once in the first trimester.

Why Are Urinary Tract Infections Common in Pregnancy?

The anatomical and physiological changes that occur during pregnancy predispose to urinary tract infection.

Progesterone-mediated smooth muscle ureteric relaxation may lead to dilatation of the upper urinary tracts; mechanical extrinsic compression of the ureters by the enlarging uterus can also produce a physiological hydroureter and hydronephrosis. The enlarged uterus can also displace the bladder superiorly and anteriorly, which may contribute to impaired bladder emptying, thereby urinary stasis and possible UTI. Finally the renal blood flow and thus the glomerular filtration rate increase by 30–40 % during pregnancy, causing enlargement and hyperemia of the kidney.

Should Asymptomatic Bacteriuria in Pregnancy Be Treated?

Yes. Studies have shown that 20–40 % of pregnant women with asymptomatic bacteriuria develop pyelonephritis during pregnancy. There is also associated significant increase in the number of low-birth-weight infants, low gestational age, and neonatal mortality.

Epidemiological evidence points to a decreased rate of pyelonephritis in pregnancy since asymptomatic bacteriuria screening became routine. In the 1970s, before screening became routine, there was a 3–4 % rate of pyelonephritis in pregnancy, compared with an incidence of 1.4 % in 2001.

A recent Cochrane review meta-analysis of trials comparing antibiotics versus no treatment for asymptomatic bacteriuria showed a substantially decreased risk of developing acute pyelonephritis.

What Are the Consequences of Not Treating a UTI in Pregnancy?

There are potential serious consequences for both mother and fetus of leaving a UTI untreated during pregnancy. Women with persistent infection despite treatment are at higher risk of delivering premature infants and development of anemia. If the UTI results in pyelonephritis, this may have the consequences listed above.

What Duration of Antibiotics Is Recommended for a UTI in Pregnancy?

Treatment of any UTI should depend on the likely antibiotic sensitivities according to local treatment guidelines.

In asymptomatic bacteriuria, there is no clear consensus as to the optimal duration of treatment. A Cochrane review analyzed studies comparing single-dose treatment with 4–7-day courses of antibiotics. There was no significant statistical difference in treatment effectiveness between the groups nor was there a conclusion as to which treatment regime was preferable.

Most symptomatic UTIs in pregnancy present as acute cystitis. A 7-day course of oral antibiotics is widely recommended, although some centers do prescribe shorter courses. Recurrent infections may be managed safely by low dose daily prophylaxis, for example, with cephalexin or nitrofurantoin.

Acute pyelonephritis has potentially serious consequences, and admission to hospital for intravenous antibiotics is recommended, although this may be converted to oral therapy after 48 h if the patient is afebrile. Initial treatment with a cephalosporin or co-amoxiclav plus aminoglycoside is recommended. A course of 10–14 days should be completed.

Which Antibiotics Should Be Avoided During Pregnancy?

Trimethoprim, a folate antagonist, has a risk of teratogenicity and should be avoided in the first trimester. Sulphonamides (risk of neonatal hemolysis and methemoglobinemia) and chloramphenicol should be avoided in the last trimester. Quinolones (e.g., ciprofloxacin) may cause arthropathy, and tetracyclines can cause dental discoloration and may also cause skeletal abnormalities. Neither should be prescribed during pregnancy (BNF).

Part II: UTI in Children

With What Signs and Symptoms Might a Child with a UTI Present?

Features of a UTI in a child may be very nonspecific. A child with an unexplained fever of over 38 °C should be tested for a UTI.

The presenting signs and symptoms vary depending on the age of the child. The most common presenting sign is a fever. Table 3.1 illustrates the variation in signs and symptoms of UTI.

Table 3.1 Symptoms and signs in infants and children with UTI

Age group		Symptoms and signs Most common ————————➤ Least common		
Infants younger than 3 months		Fever Vomiting Lethargy Irritability	Poor feeding Failure to thrive	Abdominal pain Jaundice Haematuria Offensive urine
Infants and children 3 months or older	Preverbal	Fever	Abdominal pain Loin tenderness Vomiting Poor feeding	Lethargy Irritability Haematuria Offensive urine Failure to thrive
	Verbal	Frequency Dysuria	Dysfunctional voiding Changes to continence Abdominal pain Loin tenderness	Fever Malaise Vomiting Haematuria Offensive urine Cloudy urine

How Can Urine Be Collected from Children?

Ideally a clean-catch specimen will be collected. If this is difficult, a urine collection pad can be tried. It is recommended that suprapubic aspiration should only be performed under ultrasound guidance.

If no urine can be obtained, the NICE guidelines recommend that treatment of a suspected UTI should not be delayed if there is high clinical suspicion and the child is at risk of serious illness.

How Does the Age of the Child Affect the Treatment Pathway?

The age of the child is crucial in determining their optimal management.

A child under 3 months with a suspected UTI should be immediately referred to pediatric specialist care. A urine sample must be sent for urgent microscopy and culture.

A child between the ages of 3 months and 3 years should also have urine sent off for urgent microscopy and culture. If the child has urinary tract symptoms, it is appropriate to commence antibiotic treatment while waiting for a result. However, if the child has nonspecific UTI symptoms, acute management depends on the severity of illness.

The risk of developing serious illness can be classified according to the following table suggested by NICE (Table 3.2):

If a child is deemed to be *low risk*, the urine should be sent for microscopy and culture. Treatment should commence only if cultures are positive.

Intermediate-risk patients may be referred immediately to a pediatric specialist if the situation demands. Alternatively, urgent microscopy and culture can be

Table 3.2 Traffic light system for identifying the risk of serious illness

	Green - low risk	Amber - intermediate risk	Red - high risk
Colour	• Normal colour of skin, lips and tongue	• Pallor reported by parent/carer	• Pale/mottled/ashen/blue
Activity	• Responds normally to social cues • Content/smiles • Stays awake or awakens quickly • Strong normal cry/ not crying	• Not responding normally to sodal cues • Wakes only with prolonged stimulation • Decreased activity • No smile	• No response to sodal cues • Appears ill to a healthcare professional • Unable to rouse or if roused does not stay awake • Weak, high-pitched or continuous cry

Respiratory		• Nasal flaring
		• Tachypncea:
		  – RR > 50 breaths/minute age 6 –12 months
		  – RR > 40 breaths/minute age > 12 months
		• Oxygen saturation ≤95 % in air
		• Crackles
			• Grunting
			• Tachypnoea:
			  – RR > 60 breaths/minute
			• Moderate or severe chest Indrawing

Hydration	• Normal skin and eyes • Moist mucous membranes	• Dry mucous membrane • Poor feeding In Infants • CRT ≥ 3 s • Reduced urine output	• Reduced sking turgor
Other	• None of the amber or red symptoms or signs	• Fever for ≥ 5 days • Swelling of a limb or joint • Non-weight bearing/ not using an extremity • A new lump >2 cm	• Age 0–3 months, temperature ≥ 38 °C • Age 3–6 months, temperature ≥ 39 °C • Non-blanching rash • Bulging fontanelle • Neck stiffness • Status epilepticus • Focal neurological signs • Focal seizures • Bile-stained vomiting

CRT capillary refill time
RR respiratory rate

arranged, and treatment commenced on the basis of this result. If there is no facility for immediate urine microscopy, the urine may be dipstick tested; antibiotics should be started if nitrites are present.

A *high-risk* patient should be referred immediately to a pediatric specialist. In all cases, however, urine should be sent for microscopy and culture if the child can produce a specimen.

Does Presence of Leucocytes on Dipstick Require Treatment as for a UTI?

In the absence of bacteria, leucocytes are only significant if the child has urinary tract symptoms. In this case, treatment should be initiated. Symptomatic bacteriuria always indicates a UTI and should be treated appropriately.

How Can an Upper Tract Infection/Pyelonephritis Be Differentiated from a Lower Tract Infection/Cystitis? What Treatment Is Necessary?

A bacteriuric infant or child with a temperature of greater than 38 °C and/or loin pain should be regarded as having an upper tract infection. These patients should be referred acutely to a pediatric specialist if they are deemed high risk or under 3 months of age. Otherwise, a course of low-resistance oral antibiotics for 7–10 days is recommended (e.g., a cephalosporin or co-amoxiclav).

It is recommended that lower urinary tract infections in children over 3 months are treated for 3 days with oral antibiotics. If the child remains unwell after 24–48 h, the diagnosis should be reconsidered. Antibiotic treatment should be in line with local microbiological guidance.

Which Patients with UTIs Should Undergo Acute Renal Tract Imaging?

Any infant or child with features of an atypical UTI should undergo a urinary tract ultrasound scan at the time of acute infection.

Features of an atypical UTI are one or more of:

- Abdominal or bladder mass
- Raised creatinine
- Septicemia
- Poor urine flow
- Pathogen other than *E. coli* isolated (can wait until 6 weeks for imaging if clinically well)
- Failure to respond to antibiotics within 48 h

In addition, all infants under 6 months with a first-time UTI should have an ultrasound scan of the urinary tract within 6 weeks. An infant or child with a documented atypical UTI should be referred to a local pediatric unit for consideration of a dimercaptosuccinic acid (DMSA) radionuclide scan and/or micturating cystourethrogram (MCUG).

How Is a Recurrent UTI Defined? What Investigations to These Patients Need?

A recurrent UTI is defined as either:

- *Two or more upper tract infections/pyelonephritis*
- *One upper tract infection/pyelonephritis plus one lower tract infection/cystitis*
- *Three or more lower tract infections/cystitis*

All infants and children with recurrent UTI require DMSA scanning, and those under 6 months require a MCUG. Infants with recurrent UTI should be assessed by a pediatric specialist. Recurrent UTI can result in renal scarring, progressive renal disease, and pyelonephritis.

How Common Are UTIs?

Around 8–10 % of girls and 1–3 % of boys will have had a UTI by the age of 16. Boys are affected much more commonly in the first year of life, after which the incidence falls significantly. Girls however have a higher risk of developing a UTI after the first year.

Is It True That Uncircumcised Male Infants Have a Higher Risk of Developing a UTI?

Circumcision appears to reduce the likelihood of developing a UTI by tenfold. A large meta-analysis concluded that 111 neonates being circumcised prevent one UTI in healthy males. In boys with recurrent UTI or high-grade vesicoureteric reflux, the risk of UTI recurrence is 10 and 30 % and the numbers needed to treat are 11 and 4, respectively.

Further Reading

Part I: UTI in Pregnancy

Grabe M, Bishop MC, Bjerklund Johansen TE, Botto H, et al. Urological infections. Guidelines of the European Association of Urology. 2010. EAU Guidelines Office. ISBN-13:978-90-79754-09. http://www.uroweb.org/gls/pdf/Urological%20Infections%202010.pdf.

Guinto VT, De Guia B, Festin MR, Dowswell T. Different antibiotic regimens for treating asymptomatic bacteriuria in pregnancy. Cochrane Database Syst Rev. 2010;(9): CD007855.

Lin K, Fajardo K. Screening for asymptomatic bacteriuria in adults: evidence for the U.S. Preventive Services Task Force reaffirmation recommendation statement. Ann Intern Med. 2008;149(1):W20–4.

Romero R, Oyarzun E, Mazor M, Sirtori M, et al. Meta-analysis of the relationship between asymptomatic bacteriuria and preterm delivery/low birth weight. Obstet Gynecol. 1989;73(4): 576–82.

Schnarr J, Smaill F. Asymptomatic bacteriuria and symptomatic urinary tract infections in pregnancy. Eur J Clin Invest. 2008;38 Suppl 2:50–7.

Vazquez JC, Abalos E. Treatments for symptomatic urinary tract infections during pregnancy. Cochrane Database Syst Rev. 2011;(1):CD002256.

Part II: UTI in Children

Dai B, Liu Y, Jia J, Mei C. Long-term antibiotics for the prevention of recurrent urinary tract infection in children: a systematic review and meta-analysis. Arch Dis Child. 2010;95(7):499–508.

Grabe M, Bishop MC, Bjerklund Johansen TE, Botto H, et al. Urological infections. Guidelines of the European Association of Urology. 2010. EAU Guidelines Office. ISBN-13:978-90-79754-09-0. http://www.uroweb.org/gls/pdf/Urological%20Infections%202010.pdf.

National Institute for Health and Clinical Excellence. Urinary tract infection in children; diagnosis, treatment and long-term management. CG54. London: National Institute for Health and Clinical Excellence; 2007a.

National Institute for Health and Clinical Excellence. Feverish illness in children – assessment and initial management in children younger than 5 years CG47. London: National Institute for Health and Clinical Excellence; 2007b.

Shaikh N, Morone NE, Lopez J, Chianese J, Sangvai S, D'Amico F, Hoberman A, Wald ER. Does this child have a urinary tract infection? JAMA. 2007;298(24):2895–904.

Singh-Grewal D, Macdessi J, Craig J. Circumcision for the prevention of urinary tract infection in boys: a systematic review of randomised trials and observational studies. Arch Dis Child. 2005;90(8):853–8.

Chapter 4
Tuberculosis, AIDS, and Other Uncommon Urinary Tract Infections

Andrew Symes and Abhay Rané

Abstract This chapter looks at uncommon urinary tract infections such as TB, fungal, and parasitic; it discusses the significance of conditions such as sterile pyuria and how to investigate this finding.

Keywords Uncommon • Urinary • Infections

What Is Sterile Pyuria, Is It Significant, and How Should It Be Investigated?

Sterile pyuria is the presence of significant white blood cells (WBC) in the urine, without bacteruria. It can be defined as ≥5 WBC per high-powered field (HPF) in a centrifuged specimen or >10 WBC/mm^3 of urine. Sterile pyuria is always significant and should trigger appropriate investigations to determine the possible cause, some of which are listed below:

Possible causes of sterile pyuria
Genitourinary tuberculosis (TB)
Urolithiasis
Recently treated urinary tract infection (UTI)
Urinary tract malignancy
Chlamydial urethritis
Papillary necrosis
Prostatitis
Interstitial cystitis

A. Symes, MBBS, BSc, MD, FRCS (Urol)
Department of Urology, Brighton and Sussex University Hospitals NHS Trust, Brighton, UK

A. Rané, MS, FRCS, FRCS (Urol) (✉)
Department of Urology, Surrey and Sussex Healthcare NHS Trust,
Maple House, East Surrey Hospital, Canada Avenue, Redhill, RH1 5RH, UK
e-mail: a.rane@btinternet.com

A. Rané, R. Dasgupta (eds.), *Urinary Tract Infection*
DOI 10.1007/978-1-4471-4709-1_4, © Springer-Verlag London 2013

Investigations should include a comprehensive targeted history and examination, aimed at excluding the above diagnoses. *Specific investigations should include the following, but* further, more specialized investigations should be guided by initial findings:

Midstream urine for microscopy, culture, and sensitivities
At least three early-morning urines (ideally five) for TB
A cystoscopy +/− biopsy
Upper urinary tract imaging – usually an ultrasound +/− intravenous urogram/CT scan
Urine cytology
Routine blood tests

What Is Tuberculosis, and How Does It Cause Disease?

Mycobacteria are gram-resistant, nonmotile, pleomorphic rods that are often found in habitats such as water or soil. One type is Mycobacterium tuberculosis, responsible for the development of tuberculosis (TB) in humans. It is an intracellular pathogen usually infecting mononuclear phagocytes (e.g., macrophages) and is termed an "acid-fast bacillus"; once stained, it resists decolorization with acidified organic solvents.

The World Health Organization (WHO) estimates that approximately one-third of the world's population is infected with Mycobacterium tuberculosis, with around ten million new cases per year (WHO 1997). Genitourinary TB is uncommon, accounting in the UK for only 2.6 % of all tuberculous infections [1]. The vast majority of infections are acquired through inhalation of the organism into the lungs via airborne droplet nuclei, after close contact with an actively infectious individual. Most individuals are easily able to control the initial infection and are asymptomatic, with bacilli either killed off or lying dormant.

Development of symptoms depends on both the organism and, more importantly, the host immune response, and thus, disease may occur many years later due to immunosuppression secondary to trauma, AIDS, diabetes, steroids, and other immunosuppressive agents. Prior to the advent of antibiotic therapy, the case fatality was 50 %, but this has now fallen to approximately 4 % per newly identified case.

Genitourinary TB is caused by metastatic spread of the organism through the bloodstream during the initial infection. The kidney is usually the primary organ infected with urinary disease, and other parts of the urinary tract become involved by direct extension. The initial infection occurs in the renal cortex, where the bacilli can remain dormant within granulomata for decades. This dormant infection then becomes activated due to failure of the local immune response. The primary site for infection of the genital tract is often the epididymis in men and the fallopian tubes in women, also by hematogenous spread. Similar to urinary disease, the infection then spreads to adjacent organs by direct extension.

How Does TB Present in the Urinary Tract?

TB should always be suspected in the urinary tract when a patient presents with vague, long-standing urinary symptoms without obvious cause [1]. Men are affected more commonly than women (2:1), and most patients are aged between 20 and 40 years. It is rare in children.

Infection of the kidney, ureter, and bladder usually results in urinary frequency without urgency, classically associated with sterile pyuria (not present in 20 % cases). Microscopic hematuria is also often present (50 %), but visible hematuria is rare (10 %). Symptoms are often intermittent and pain is rare, although recurrent cystitis may be an early warning sign.

Recurrent hematospermia is a rare presenting symptom, but tuberculous epididymitis may be the first and only presenting symptom of genitourinary TB, which may involve the testis by direct extension. Clinically it is often identical to acute epididymo-orchitis, with a painful, inflamed scrotal swelling.

How Should the Diagnosis Be Confirmed?

The tuberculin test involves intradermal injection of a purified protein derivative of tuberculin, which, when positive, causes an inflammatory reaction at the site. A positive reaction only signifies previous infection and is not synonymous with active infection. Diagnosis therefore relies on urine examination.

Sterile pyuria is the classic urine analysis finding with microscopic hematuria present 50 % of the time. Routine urine culture may show secondary bacterial infection (20 %); however, cultures for *M. tuberculosis* take 6–8 weeks, as the organism is slow growing. As the organism is only intermittently excreted, at least three early morning urine specimens (pooled over night) should be sent and inoculated on Lowenstein-Jensen culture media.

The Ziehl-Neelsen stain used diagnostically on sputum, however, is not commonly employed in urine due to false positives. More recently a polymerase chain reaction method on pooled urine samples has been developed and appears to offer sensitivity and specificity of 96 and 98 %, respectively [2].

Imaging has an important role to play in diagnosis. Intravenous urogram, or more commonly CT urogram, can be used to provide functional information about:

1. Renal lesions – infundibular stenosis, calyceal and parenchymal destruction, and calcification.
2. Ureters – strictures and dilatation and the condition of the bladder wall.
3. Cystoscopy and biopsy are not essential tests in diagnosing genitourinary TB but are often employed in ruling out other conditions such as malignancy.

What Complications Does TB Infection Cause in the Urinary Tract?

Renal

Caseating granulomata occur in the kidney, and when healing occurs, fibrous tissue is left with calcium deposition resulting in calcified lesions. If extensive this may lead to parenchymal destruction and even "autonephrectomy" [3]. In addition calyceal strictures, papillary necrosis, and ureteropelvic junction obstruction may occur.

Ureter

In a similar process strictures may occur anywhere in the ureter causing obstruction. Most commonly these occur at the vesicoureteric junction.

Bladder

Lesions are initially centered around the ureteric orifice and may be discrete ulcers or inflamed edematous tissue. If untreated they may become extensive, resulting in a fibrotic and contracted bladder.

Epididymis

Infection of the epididymis presents as an epididymo-orchitis and sometimes even as a fistula.

How Is TB Treated?

Treatment of active *M. tuberculosis* infection is with a combination of antituberculous drugs such as isoniazid, rifampicin, streptomycin, pyrazinamide, and ethambutol. Multidrug therapy aims to diminish the likelihood of drug-resistant organisms developing. Therapy is continued for 6 months in most cases [4]. The role of surgery has declined with the successes of medical treatment and is now largely centered on organ preservation and reconstruction, as opposed to excision [5]. It is usually delayed until at least 4–6 weeks of medical therapy has been administered.

What Is AIDS and How Is It Diagnosed?

Acquired immunodeficiency syndrome (AIDS) refers to the disorder caused by HIV (human immunodeficiency virus) infection. HIV is a retrovirus that infects and kills T-helper cells, one of the body's main cellular defenses against infection. HIV is spread through contact with blood, semen, and vaginal secretions – for example, by sexual intercourse, use of contaminated needles or blood products, or from mother to baby during childbirth.

The course of HIV infection is very variable and typically occurs over 8–12 years [6]. *Three distinct phases exist*:

1. Primary infection – a self-limiting syndrome lasting less than 14 days and mimicking many acute febrile illnesses.
2. Chronic asymptomatic infection – lasting around 10 years.
3. Overt AIDS – defined by the development of serious opportunistic infections, neoplasms, or other life-threatening conditions resulting from immunosuppression caused by HIV infection. It usually occurs when CD4$^+$ counts fall below 200 cells/mm^3 and leads to death within 2–3 years if untreated.

Standardized laboratory assays are available for HIV testing and screening for HIV antibodies using an enzyme-linked immunosorbent assay (ELISA). Testing is a two-step process, with the initial screening assay retested to exclude laboratory error. If positive, a confirmatory assay is also performed to confirm the diagnosis [6].

What Are the Urological Complications of HIV/AIDS

The two most common sequelae of AIDS are infections and malignancy; however, numerous other complications can occur. These are summarized in the table below.

Infections	
Genitourinary tuberculosis	Papillary necrosis, autonephrectomy, strictures
Renal	CMV, aspergillosis, toxoplasmosis
Penile and urethral	Genital herpes, warts, pelvic inflammatory disease, Reiter's disease (uveitis, arthritis, urethritis)
Prostate	Prostatitis (common organisms + fungal, TB)
Testis and epididymis	Epididymo-orchitis (common organisms + fungal, TB)
Syphilis	Resurgent in the UK
Fournier's gangrene	Fulminant necrotizing fasciitis of scrotum
UTIs	Usual urinary tract pathogens, e.g., *E. coli*
Malignancy	
Kaposi's sarcoma	Assoc with herpes virus infection, genital skin
Squamous cell carcinoma	Also assoc with HPV infection, penile or genital skin
Testicular cancer	50× increased risk of germ cell and non-germ cell tumors
Non-Hodgkin's lymphoma	Lymph nodes primarily but can be genitourinary organs/genital skin

Renal dysfunction and/or failure	
HIV-associated nephropathy	Proteinuria and renal insufficiency/end-stage renal failure
Stones	
Protease inhibitors	Indinavir/atazanavir
	Radiolucent and may not be seen on CT
	Management is temporary cessation of drug with hydration
Voiding dysfunction	
Voiding dysfunction	Most common is urinary retention 54 %, detrusor overactivity 27 %, bladder outflow obstruction 18 %
Erectile dysfunction/infertility	
Erectile dysfunction	Worsen as disease progresses. HIV infection is also cytotoxic to sertoli/germ cells – testicular atrophy
Infertility	Abnormal semen parameters assoc with testicular atrophy. Risk of HIV transmission

Should Men Be Routinely Circumcised to Reduce Risk of HIV Transmission?

Three prospective randomized clinical trials of adult male circumcision in South Africa, Kenya, and Uganda reported highly significant reductions in risk of HIV infection among participants randomly assigned to circumcision [7–9], and indeed, the trials were stopped early in some cases due to the overwhelming demonstration of the significant advantage for the circumcised group. This is mirrored by a meta-analysis of studies that demonstrated a highly significant reduced risk of HIV infection in circumcised men [10].

Despite this strong evidence, the issue remains contentious, as many would argue that in the UK, the relatively low rates of HIV in non-high-risk populations do not justify the invasive nature of the procedure and may indeed encourage risky behavior (i.e., lack of condom use).

What Is Schistosomiasis and Its Life Cycle?

Schistosomiasis is a chronic disease caused by parasitic infection with schistosomes, parasitic trematodes. Paired adult male and female worms reside in the venous plexuses of the abdominal viscera. *S. haematobium* worms live mainly in the venous plexuses around the bladder and are responsible for urinary schistosomiasis. Other types will not be discussed here. *S. haematobium* worms are endemic to tropical areas of Southeast Asia, Africa, South America, the Middle East, and the Caribbean, with 80–90 million persons infected. Of these, up to 40 million people have complications secondary to the disease.

The life cycle of *S. haematobium* is complex and can be divided into an asexual, snail phase and a sexual, human phase (see text and figure below).

Snail phase – asexual

- Free swimming miracidium enters snail.
- Becomes sporocyst (one miracidium makes 40 sporocysts).
- Each sporocyst forms ~400 active parasites called cercariae – released into water.

Human phase – sexual

- Cercariae penetrate skin to become schistosomulum in liver.
- Adults pair up and move to bladder vesical veins.
- Copulate 3–6 years, ~500 eggs/day.
- Eggs migrate into bladder, penetrate mucosa, and flush out miracidium larvae.

Schistosomiasis Life Cycle (**CDC/Alexander J. da Silva, PhD/Melanie Moser**)

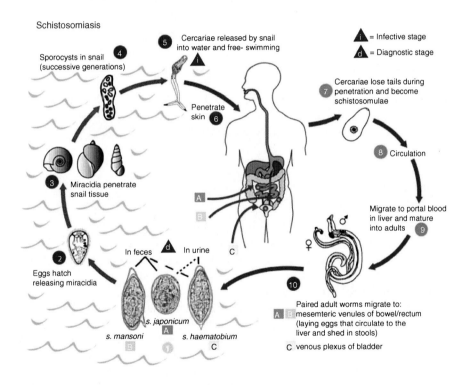

What Are the Clinical Manifestations of Schistosomiasis, and How Is It Diagnosed and Treated?

Clinically, schistosomiasis can be divided into an active and chronic phase. Active infection, Katayama fever, is rare among endemic populations and is more commonly seen in noninfected travelers. It may result in fever, lymphadenopathy, splenomegaly, and urticaria [11].

Chronic schistosomiasis is much more common and has several different manifestations. The classical initial clinical presentation is hematuria with terminal dysuria. This can be severe enough to produce anemia and clot retention [12]. Next, patients enter a chronic active phase where symptoms are largely related to a contracted bladder and consist of pelvic pain, urgency, frequency, and urinary incontinence. During this phase, the ureters may become obstructed resulting in hydroureteronephrosis. Finally, the chronic inactive phase is where the infection has burnt out and symptoms result from complications, such as nonfunctioning obstructed kidneys.

The diagnosis is made in a patient who has had exposure to an endemic area. The presence of terminally spined eggs in the urine is diagnostic of active *S. haematobium* infection. As excretion peaks between 10 a.m. and 2 p.m., a midday urine is sent for microscopy. If eggs are not seen, either bladder or rectal mucosal biopsy may show the presence of eggs, with cystoscopy often reported as showing sandy patches. In the inactive form of the disease, eggs are not excreted, and the diagnosis is made radiographically. Plain X-ray may show a calcified bladder, with calcification seen anywhere along the urinary tract. CT or IVU may help diagnose ureteric obstruction, strictures, and nonfunctioning kidneys.

Praziquantel is the drug of choice for treatment of schistosomiasis. Cure rates approach 100 % and it is given in two divided oral doses of 40 mg/kg. Side effects are mild and self-limiting. Surgery is now reserved for complications that have not resolved after medical therapy (e.g., ureteric obstruction).

What Fungal Infections of the Urinary Tract Are You Aware of?

With the exception of Candida species, the urinary tract is rarely involved in fungal infections. Rare diseases, such as aspergillosis, cryptococcus, histoplasmosis, and coccidioidomycosis, may involve the urinary tract but are often part of disseminated disease in immunocompromised patients.

Candida albicans is responsible for the majority of fungal infections in the urinary tract. The number of these infections has risen dramatically with the increasing use of broad-spectrum antibiotics, indwelling vascular and urinary catheters, and immunosuppressants. Candidal infection is commonly seen on the penis, vulva and vagina, and on the skin around stomas. The majority of patients with candiduria are asymptomatic, although emphysematous cystitis has been seen in diabetic patients with candida. Infection of the upper urinary tract with candida can also occur and may present like acute pyelonephritis. Infection can arise either through hematogenous spread in systemic infection or via ascendance from the lower urinary tract. Renal abscesses, pyelonephritis, urinary obstruction, and fungal balls requiring surgical removal can all occur. Diagnosis is made by direct microscopy of urine, with cultures usually unhelpful. Radiographic imaging is directed at identifying complications.

Candiduria may reflect contamination or colonization, but persistence requires evaluation and consideration of treatment [13]. Not all patients require treatment, and in many instances, removal of a catheter or discontinuation of antibiotic therapy may be enough to clear the infection [14]. Patients who are undergoing urinary tract instrumentation should, however, be treated. Systemic treatment with oral or intravenous fluconazole achieves high urinary concentration and is the first line if treatment is required. Intravenous amphotericin has also been used in difficult to treat infections but comes at the price of toxicity. Local irrigation with antifungals to bladders and kidneys via catheters and nephrostomies has also been used with varying degrees of success.

What Is Emphysematous Pyelitis/Pyelonephritis?

Emphysematous pyelitis is an infection of the renal collecting system by gas-forming bacteria. It is often associated with diabetes mellitus (50 %) and, if untreated, has a mortality of up to 20 %. It presents in a similar fashion to acute pyelonephritis, with systemic symptoms and loin pain, and is often preceded by lower urinary tract symptoms such as cystitis. Management involves fluid resuscitation, intravenous antibiotics, strict diabetic control, and if necessary, urinary tract drainage via retrograde ureteric stenting or nephrostomy.

Emphysematous pyelonephritis is an acute, severe, necrotizing infection of the renal parenchyma and perirenal tissue, which results in the presence of gas within the renal parenchyma, collecting system, or perinephric tissue. It is associated with diabetes 90 % of the time and has a mortality of 50 %. Presentation is of an acutely unwell septic patient, often with poorly controlled diabetes or even as a diabetic ketoacidosis. The management is along ABC principles and should be considered as a surgical emergency. Broad-spectrum antibiotics and tight diabetic control is essential, and these patients often require emergency nephrectomy.

Emphysematous pyelonephritis is different to xanthogranulomatous pyelonephritis which is a chronic severe infection leading to destruction of renal tissue and eventually resulting in a nonfunctioning kidney. It is usually seen with upper urinary tract obstruction and stones and may be difficult to distinguish from renal cell carcinoma on CT scanning, thus often ending up in a nephrectomy.

How Do You Manage a Systemically Unwell Diabetic with Cellulitis of the Scrotum?

This patient should be seen immediately and an assessment made along ABC principles. He should be admitted to hospital and fully resuscitated with oxygen and IV fluids and should also be given broad-spectrum intravenous antibiotics, as guided by local microbiological advice. Blood tests should be sent off for renal function, glucose, full blood count, C-reactive protein, and clotting. Diabetics who have a source of illness, especially sepsis, are at increased risk of developing diabetic keto-acidosis, and in that instance, a sliding scale should be commenced to control blood sugar. He should be regularly reviewed, and if any clinical signs of deterioration present, then early involvement of ITU/HDU is essential. With scrotal cellulitis, there is no role for surgical management. If the diagnosis were unclear, an urgent ultrasound of the scrotum would help rule out an underlying abscess requiring drainage.

What Is Fournier's Gangrene, and How Is It Treated?

Fournier's gangrene is a polymicrobial necrotizing fasciitis of the perianal, perineal, or genital areas. The bacteria involved act synergistically to invade and destroy fascial planes and are composed of aerobes (e.g., *E. coli*) and anaerobes (e.g., bacteroides). Predisposing factors include diabetes, alcoholism, steroids, malnutrition, and HIV infection. Trauma, recent surgery, and the presence of foreign bodies may be inciting events, and causative factors are found in more than 75 % of cases. It often starts insidiously and extreme pain is an early finding along with systemic upset. As the disease progresses, skin overlying the affected region becomes discolored, eventually becoming gangrenous. Crepitus may be present, and by this stage, the patient usually shows signs of severe sepsis or even septic shock.

Fournier's gangrene is a true surgical emergency necessitating radical debridement in theater, which is often repeated at second look 24–48 h later. Urinary and fecal diversion may be required depending on the source of infection. Broad-spectrum antibiotic cover is given with aggressive resuscitation, usually on a high-dependency/intensive care unit. Once the infection has settled, these patients often require plastic surgery consultation to cover the large defects left by debridement. Mortality from this condition can be as high as 75 % [15].

Key Points
- Sterile pyuria is a significant finding and should trigger appropriate investigations. It may be the only presenting sign of genitourinary tuberculosis.
- Genitourinary TB is uncommon and usually arises through hematogenous spread first to the kidney and then down through the urinary tract.
- Genitourinary TB should be suspected in any patient with vague, poorly defined, long-standing urinary symptoms without an obvious cause.
- Diagnosis of urinary tract TB requires at least three early-morning urine specimens; however, pooled urinary PCR may speed up diagnosis.

- AIDS sufferers can manifest numerous differing urinary tract symptoms, but generally infections, which may be atypical, and malignancies are the most common.
- Circumcision significantly reduces the risk of HIV transmission but is controversial, and not part of current UK practice.
- Schistosomiasis is a parasitic infection not endemic to the UK. It has a complex life cycle involving humans and snails.
- Candidal urinary tract infections are associated with immunocompromise, either systemic or through breach of natural host defense mechanisms, e.g., urinary catheter.
- Candida does not always require treatment; with cessation of antibiotics sometimes, this is all that is required to terminate the infection.
- Emphysematous pyelitis/pyelonephritis, scrotal cellulitis, and Fournier's gangrene are rare urinary tract infections, but potentially life-threatening and require urgent urological referral and management.

References

1. Garcia-Rodriguez JA, Garcia Sanchez JE, Munoz Bellido JL, et al. Genitourinary tuberculosis in Spain: review of 81 cases. Clin Infect Dis. 1994;18:557–61.
2. Moussa OM, Eraky I, El-Far MA, Osman HG, Ghoneim MA. Rapid diagnosis of genitourinary tuberculosis by polymerase chain reaction and non-radioactive DNA hybridization. J Urol. 2000;164:584–8.
3. Wong SH, Lau WY. The surgical management of non-functioning tuberculous kidneys. J Urol. 1980;124:187–91.
4. Iseman MD. A clinician's guide to tuberculosis. Philadelphia: Lippincott Williams and Wilkins. 2006.
5. Mochalova TP, Starikov IY. Reconstructive surgery for treatment of urogenital tuberculosis: 30 years of observation. World J Surg. 1997;21:511–5.
6. Cohen J, Powderly W. Infectious diseases: 2-volume set (infectious diseases (Armstrong/Mosby)). Edinburgh/New York: Mosby; 2003.
7. Auvert B, Taljaard D, Lagarde E, Sobngwi-Tambekou J, Sitta R, Puren A. Randomized, controlled intervention trial of male circumcision for reduction of HIV infection risk: the ANRS 1265 Trial. PLoS Med. 2005;2:e298.
8. Bailey RC, Moses S, Parker CB, et al. Male circumcision for HIV prevention in young men in Kisumu, Kenya: a randomised controlled trial. Lancet. 2007;369:643–56.
9. Gray RH, Kigozi G, Serwadda D, et al. Male circumcision for HIV prevention in men in Rakai, Uganda: a randomised trial. Lancet. 2007;369:657–66.
10. Weiss HA, Quigley MA, Hayes RJ. Male circumcision and risk of HIV infection in sub-Saharan Africa: a systematic review and meta-analysis. AIDS. 2000;14:2361–70.
11. de Jesus AR, Silva A, Santana LB, et al. Clinical and immunologic evaluation of 31 patients with acute schistosomiasis mansoni. J Infect Dis. 2002;185:98–105.
12. Wilkins HA, Goll PH, Moore PJ. Schistosoma haematobium infection and haemoglobin concentrations in a Gambian community. Ann Trop Med Parasitol. 1985;79:159–61.
13. Pappas PG, Rex JH, Sobel JD, et al. Guidelines for treatment of candidiasis. Clin Infect Dis. 2004;38:161–89.

14. Kauffman CA, Vazquez JA, Sobel JD, et al. Prospective multicenter surveillance study of funguria in hospitalized patients. The National Institute for Allergy and Infectious Diseases (NIAID) Mycoses Study Group. Clin Infect Dis. 2000;30:14–8.
15. Czymek R, Hildebrand P, Kleemann M, et al. New insights into the epidemiology and etiology of Fournier's gangrene: a review of 33 patients. Infection. 2009;37:306–12.

Chapter 5
Urinary Tract Infection in Diabetic Patients

Taufiq Shaikh and Ranan Dasgupta

Abstract Certain groups of patient are at higher risk of UTI, for example, diabetics. We discuss the reasons why they are more prone in this chapter. We also touch upon the more severe complications, which the reader should be aware of, such as emphysematous pyelonephritis. Some of these cases require urgent surgery, and therefore it is essential that the clinician has a low threshold of suspicion in cases of urosepsis in diabetics, and therefore early involvement of urological input is justified.

Keywords Diabetic • Diabetes mellitus • Urinary tract infection • Emphysematous pyelonephritis • Papillary necrosis

Are UTIs More Common in Diabetics?

UTI is one of the most common infections in diabetic patients. Patients with diabetes have an increased risk of urinary tract infection as compared to nondiabetic population [1]. This is true for both asymptomatic bacteriuria (ASB) and symptomatic UTI.

The rate of asymptomatic bacteriuria is three to four times higher in diabetic women as compared to nondiabetic women [2, 3]. However, there is not much difference in the prevalence of asymptomatic bacteriuria in diabetic and nondiabetic men [4]. The relative risk of symptomatic UTI in diabetics is about 1.39–1.43 times more as compared to nondiabetics [5].

T. Shaikh
Charing Cross Hospital, Imperial College Healthcare NHS Trust,
Fulham Palace Road, London, W6 8RF, UK

R. Dasgupta, MBBChir, MA, MD, FRCS (Urol) (✉)
Department of Urology, Imperial College Healthcare NHS Trust,
St Mary's Hospital, Praed Street, London W2 1NY, UK
e-mail: ranandg@yahoo.co.uk

A. Rané, R. Dasgupta (eds.), *Urinary Tract Infection*,
DOI 10.1007/978-1-4471-4709-1_5, © Springer-Verlag London 2013

What Course Does UTI Run in Diabetic Patients?

In diabetic patients, UTI has a higher chance to run a complicated course as compared to nondiabetic patients. Diabetes predisposes to more severe infections which are difficult to treat and recur more often. The chances of bacteremia and need for hospital admission also are higher in diabetic patients with UTI.

What Is the Pathogenesis of Development of UTI in Diabetic Patients?

As in nondiabetic patients, the essential step in the pathogenesis of UTI is the adherence of pathogenic microbes to the bladder mucosal lining. In most gram-negative uropathogens, this is achieved by various virulence factors such as H antigen, fimbriae, or adhesins. In the case of *E. coli* (the most commonly studied organism), virulence factors are fimbriae. Type 1 fimbriae bind to glycoprotein receptors in uroepithelium, whereas Type 2 fimbriae bind to glycolipid receptors in the kidney [6].

Once the bacteria are bound, urothelial cells internalize bacteria by an active process similar to endocytosis and require tyrosine phosphorylation [7]. This is followed by an inflammatory response from the host immune system. The inflammatory response consists of steps involving uroepithelial cell activation associated with transmembrane signaling, resulting in the production of distinct inflammatory mediators. Usually, this is followed by the direction of the innate immune cells to the infectious focus which leads to local destruction and elimination of the invading bacteria [6]. This process involves the complement system, Toll-like receptors (TLRs), urinary Tamm-Horsfall proteins (THPs), cytokines, and adhesion molecules [8]. Bacteria can also invade uroepithelium where they replicate and form quiescent intracellular reservoirs, which may serve as a possible source for recurrent UTIs.

What Is the Reason for Higher Prevalence of UTI in Diabetics?

The presence of glucosuria and impairment of the granulocyte function in the diabetic patients, although long suggested as the reason for increased risk of UTI, have not been conclusively proven in vivo [9–11]. Some studies have suggested that decreased urinary levels of IL-6 and IL-8 in diabetic patients contribute to increased incidence of UTI [12]. It has also been suggested that there is increased adherence of bacteria to the urothelium in diabetic patients. This is due to decreased ability of THP to bind type 1 fimbriated organisms, possibly because of an additional glycosylation of THP in diabetic patients, and a positive correlation with poorly controlled diabetes [13, 14].

What Are the Risk Factors That Predispose to UTI in Diabetes Mellitus (DM)?

As in nondiabetic patients, host factors tend to be either urinary tract obstruction, stasis, reflux, instrumentation, or sexual intercourse [9]. Additional factors in diabetic patients that might predispose them to UTI include age, glycemic control, duration of DM, diabetic cystopathy, frequent hospitalization, vaginitis, and vascular complications [15].

What Is the Clinical Presentation and in What Way Can It Present Differently?

The clinical presentation of UTI in diabetic patients can range from asymptomatic bacteriuria to severe life-threatening sepsis. The incidence of symptomatic UTI in the form of dysuria, frequency, abdominal discomfort, and urgency is higher in diabetic patients [15]. Occasionally, UTI in this group of patients might also be associated with hematuria.

In diabetic patients, there are increased chances of UTI running a complicated course and presenting with acute pyelonephritis. The risk of hospital admission for acute pyelonephritis can increase 20–30 times in diabetic patients less than 44 years of age. The risk is 30–50 times in diabetics over 44 years of age [16]. Bilateral pyelonephritis is more common in diabetic patients [17]. Papillary necrosis, renal abscess, emphysematous pyelonephritis, and systemic sepsis may also occur [18].

What Is Emphysematous UTI?

Emphysematous UTI is a severe necrotizing infection and, as the name suggests, it is characterized by gas formation along the urinary tract. It mainly can be in the form of emphysematous pyelonephritis or emphysematous cystitis. Emphysematous pyelonephritis (EPN) can involve the collecting system, renal parenchyma, and the perirenal tissues, whereas emphysematous cystitis involves the bladder wall. The infection has a severe and fulminant course and can be life-threatening if not recognized and treated early. Gas formation is thought to occur as a result of mixed acid fermentation of glucose [19]. A high degree of suspicion is required for diagnosis, which is made by a radiological demonstration of gas formation along the renal tract. A CT KUB is the investigation of choice and delineates the localization or the extent of gas formation, thus helping formulate an optimal management plan [20].

Treatment comprises active resuscitation, electrolyte and blood glucose monitoring, and correction and administration of antibiotics targeting gram-negative bacteria. Any associated obstruction along the urinary tract, if present, should be relieved, and if there is extensive gas formation with renal destruction, a nephrectomy may be warranted [21].

What Is Renal Papillary Necrosis?

Renal papillary necrosis is an important complication of UTI in diabetics. Symptoms include chills, fever, and acute renal insufficiency. The pathogenesis is not well understood but is presumed to be due to the marginal vascular supply at the papilla, which becomes further compromised by infection, leading to infarction and sloughing of the papillae [22].

What Are the Main Organisms Implicated for UTI in Diabetes, and Is There Any Difference Compared to UTI in Nondiabetics?

The causative microorganisms of UTIs in patients with DM are similar to those found in nondiabetic patients with complicated UTI. The same is true for the antibiotic resistance and sensitivity patterns [23]. The most common causative organism for UTI is *E. coli*. Other pathogenic microbes include *Klebsiella* sp., Group B streptococci, *Enterococcus* spp., and Pseudomonas. Diabetes mellitus, per se, is not considered to be a risk factor for the development of antibiotic resistance.

Should ASB Be Treated in Diabetics?

ASB is a risk factor for symptomatic UTI in nondiabetic patient population [24] and increases the risk of recurrent UTI, progressive renal failure, and hypertension [25]. The limited number of studies in diabetic patients show that ASB increases the risk of symptomatic UTI in type II diabetics, as compared to type I diabetics [26]. There is no relationship between ASB and deterioration in renal function [27], as was previously thought [26]. The risk of complications is not reduced by antimicrobial therapy of ASB and, therefore, should not be an indication to screen for or treat ASB [28].

Is the Treatment of UTI in DM Different from Nondiabetics and What Important, or Special, Considerations Should Be Given to Such Patients?

As the causative microbes and their antimicrobial sensitivity in diabetics are similar to nondiabetic patients, the choice of antimicrobial treatment should be similar and based on the local resistance patterns of the common uropathogens [29]. Treatment protocols should avoid nephrotoxic agents as much as possible. A 2-week treatment regime is as effective as a 6-week regime. Any recurrence seen 4–8 weeks after treatment is a reinfection rather than a relapse [30].

Even though there is no general agreement, UTI in diabetics is treated as "complicated" by most clinicians [31, 32]. Preferred drugs are fluoroquinolones and amoxicillin-clavulanic acid, which achieve high levels in urine and urinary tissues on administration [33]. Trimethoprim/sulfamethoxazole is usually avoided as it can lead to hypoglycemia [34].

Although evidence is lacking, the duration of antimicrobial therapy is longer (7–14 days) than in the nondiabetic population, particularly with frequent upper tract involvement and increased risk of serious complications. The treatment of uncomplicated pyelonephritis does not differ from that of nondiabetic patient group. In these cases, a 7-day regime of oral fluoroquinolones is considered to be a better choice than 2 weeks of trimethoprim [35]. For more severe infections requiring hospital admission and those with sepsis, a combination of intravenous agents based on local policy need to be administered. These agents include fluoroquinolones, aminoglycosides, ceftriaxones, Tazocin, and meropenems.

For recurrent symptomatic infections, such as those in nondiabetics, antibiotic prophylaxis can be initiated in diabetic group as well.

What Non-antimicrobial and Preventative Strategies Can Be Adopted by Such Patients?

The non-antimicrobial strategies to prevent UTI are essentially similar to those that help in prevention of UTI in the nondiabetic patient group. General advice includes sufficient fluid intake, complete emptying of the bladder, less frequent use of catheters, and avoidance of spermicides in women [36]. Other strategies include ingestion of cranberry juice [37, 38] and oral or vaginal administration of lactobacillus [39]. Cranberry tablets are considered a better alternative to cranberry juice in diabetic patients. Estrogen administration can be beneficial in the reduction of recurrence rates of UTI in postmenopausal diabetic women [40]. Two types of vaccines for prevention of UTI have been developed, but both have been withdrawn; although safe, these vaccines were effective in only about a third of patients they were administered to.

Key Points
- Diabetic patients are at higher risk of developing a UTI.
- UTI has a higher risk of complications, and in diabetics, involvement of the upper tract requiring hospital admission is greater.
- The complications to carefully be aware of include emphysematous pyelonephritis, renal papillary necrosis, renal abscess, and septicemia.
- The most common causative organism for UTI in diabetics is *E. coli*.

- Asymptomatic bacteriuria is not an indication for antimicrobial treatment in diabetics.
- The choice of antibiotics should be based on local resistance and sensitivity patterns and does not differ much from the nondiabetic group.
- Antibiotic prophylaxis can be initiated in patients with recurrent UTIs.
- Nephrotoxic antimicrobials should be avoided in diabetic patients.
- Cranberry tablets are considered a better alternative to cranberry juice in diabetic patients.

References

1. Muller LM, et al. Increased risk of common infections in patients with type 1 and type 2 diabetes. Clin Infect Dis. 2005;41:281–8.
2. Zhanel GG, Harding GK, Nicolle LE. Asymptomatic bacteriuria in patients with diabetes mellitus. Rev Infect Dis. 1991;13(1):150–4.
3. Geerlings SE, Stolk RP, Camps MJL, et al. Asymptomatic bacteriuria may be considered a complication in women with diabetes. Diabetes Care. 2000;23(6):744–9.
4. Forland M, Thomas V, Shelokov A. Urinary tract infections in patients with diabetes mellitus. Studies on antibody coating of bacteria. JAMA. 1977;238(18):1924–6.
5. Shah BR, Hux JE. Quantifying the risk of infectious diseases for people with diabetes. Diabetes Care. 2003;26:510–3.
6. Mulvey MA, Schiling JD, Martinez JJ, Hultgren SJ. Bad bugs and beleaguered bladders. Interplay between uropathogenic Escherichia coli and innate host defenses. Proc Natl Acad Sci USA. 2000;97:8829–35.
7. Palmer LM, Reilly TJ, Utsalo SJ, Donnenberg MS. Internalization of E coli by human renal epithelial cells is associated with tyrosine phosphorylation of specific host proteins. Infect Immun. 1997;65:2570–5.
8. Mak RH, Kuo HJ. Pathogenesis of urinary tract infection: an update. Curr Opin Pediatr. 2006;18(2):148–52.
9. Geerlings SE, Stolk RP, Camps MJL, et al. Risk factors for symptomatic urinary tract infection in women with diabetes mellitus. Diabetes Care. 2000;23(12):1737–41.
10. Delamaire M, Maugendre D, Moreno M, et al. Impaired leukocyte functions in diabetic patients. Diabet Med. 1997;14(1):29–34.
11. Balasoiu D, Van Kessel KC, Van Kats-Renaud HJ, et al. Granulocyte function in women with diabetes and asymptomatic bacteriuria. Diabetes Care. 1997;20(3):392–5.
12. Geerlings SE, Brouwer EC, Van Kessel KCPM, et al. Cytokine secretion is impaired in women with diabetes mellitus. Eur J Clin Invest. 2000;30(11):995–1001.
13. Geerlings SE, Meiland R, Van Lith EC, et al. Adherence of type 1-fimbriated Escherichia coli to uroepithelial cells: more in diabetic women than in controls. Diabetes Care. 2002;25:1405–9.
14. Geerlings SE. Urinary tract infections in patients with diabetes mellitus: epidemiology, pathogenesis and treatment. Int J Antimicrob Agents. 2008;31 Suppl 1:S54–7.
15. Patterson JE, Andriole VT. Bacterial urinary tract infections in diabetes. Infect Dis Clin North Am. 1997;11(3):735–50.
16. Nicolle LE, Friesen D, Harding GK, et al. Hospitalization for acute pyelonephritis in Manitoba, Canada, during the period from 1989 to 1992, impact of diabetes, pregnancy, and aboriginal origin. Clin Infect Dis. 1996;22(6):1051–6.
17. Calvet HM, Yoshikawa TT. Infections in diabetes. Infect Dis Clin North Am. 2001;15(2):407–21.
18. Wheat LJ. Infection and diabetes mellitus. Diabetes Care. 1980;3(1):187–97.

19. Huang JJ, Chen KW, Ruaan MK. Mixed acid fermentation of glucose as a mechanism of emphysematous urinary tract infection. J Urol. 1991;146(1):148–51.
20. Wan YL, Lee TY, Bullard MJ, et al. Acute gas producing bacterial renal infection: correlation between imaging findings and clinical outcome. Radiology. 1996;198:433–8.
21. Pontin AR, Barnes RD, Medscape. Current management of emphysematous pyelonephritis. Nat Rev Urol. 2009;6(5):272–9.
22. Griffin MD, Bergstralhn EJ, Larson TS. Renal papillary necrosis – a sixteen-year clinical experience. J Am Soc Nephrol. 1995;6:248–56.
23. Bonadio M, Costarelli S, Morelli G, Tartaglia T. The influence of diabetes mellitus on the spectrum of uropathogens and the antimicrobial resistance in elderly adult patients with urinary tract infection. BMC Infect Dis. 2006;6:54.
24. Hooton TM, Scholes D, Stapleton AE, et al. A prospective study of asymptomatic bacteriuria in sexually active young women. N Engl J Med. 2000;343(14):992–7.
25. Ronald AR, Patullo LS. The natural history of urinary infections in adults. Infect Dis Clin North Am. 1991;75(2):299–312.
26. Geerlings SE, Stolk RP, Camps MJL, et al. Consequences of asymptomatic bacteriuria in women with diabetes mellitus. Arch Intern Med. 2001;161(11):1421–7.
27. Meiland R, Geerlings SE, Stolk RP, Netten PM, Schneeberger PM, Hoepelman IM. Asymptomatic bacteriuria in women with diabetes mellitus: effect on renal function after 6 years follow-up. Arch Intern Med. 2006;166:2222–7.
28. Harding GK, Zhanel GG, Nicolle LE, Cheang M. Manitoba diabetes urinary tract infection study group. Antimicrobial treatment in diabetic women with asymptomatic bacteriuria. N Engl J Med. 2003;348:957–8.
29. Meiland R, Geerlings SE, De Neeling AJ, Hoepelman AI. Diabetes mellitus in itself is not a risk factor for antibiotic resistance in Escherichia coli isolated from patients with bacteriuria. Diabet Med. 2004;21:1032–4.
30. Forland M, Thomas VL. The treatment of urinary tract infections in women with diabetes mellitus. Diabetes Care. 1985;8(5):499–506.
31. Melekos MD, Naber KG. Complicated urinary tract infections. Int J Antimicrob Agents. 2000;15(4):247–56.
32. Ronald A, Ludwig E. Urinary tract infections in adults with diabetes. Int J Antimicrob Agents. 2001;17(4):287–92.
33. Schaeffer AJ. Bacterial urinary tract infections in diabetes. J Urol. 1998;160(1):293.
34. Poretsky L, Moses AC. Hypoglycemia associated with trimethoprim/sulfamethoxazole therapy. Diabetes Care. 1984;7:508–9.
35. Talan DA, Stamm WE, Hooton TM, Moran GJ, Burke T, Iravani A, et al. Comparison of ciprofloxacin (7 days) and trimethoprim-sulfamethoxazole (14 days) in acute uncomplicated pyelonephritis in women. JAMA. 2000;283:1583–90.
36. Stapleton A, Stamm WE. Prevention of urinary tract infection. Infect Dis Clin North Am. 1997;11:719–34.
37. Lowe FC, Fagelman E. Cranberry juice and urinary tract infections: what is the evidence? Urology. 2001;57(3):407–13.
38. Kontiokari T, Sundqvist K, Nuutinen M, et al. Randomised trial of cranberry-lingonberry juice and Lactobacillus GG drink for the prevention of urinary tract infections in women. BMJ. 2001;322(7302):1571–3.
39. Boris S, Suarez JE, Vazquez F, et al. Adherence of human vaginal lactobacilli to vaginal epithelial cells and interaction with uropathogens. Infect Immun. 1998;66(5):1985–9.
40. Hextall A. Oestrogens and lower urinary tract function. Maturitas. 2000;36(2):83–92.

Chapter 6
Catheter-Associated Urinary Tract Infections

Uwais Bashir Mufti and Ranan Dasgupta

This chapter is based on the European and Asian Guidelines on Management and Prevention of Catheter-associated Urinary Tract Infections.

Abstract One of the difficulties with indwelling catheters is the propensity to develop catheter-related infections. While drainage of the bladder ensures a low-pressure reservoir (protecting the upper tracts and also designed to reduce the frequency of infections), unfortunately colonization of the catheter with a biofilm leads to urinary infection. The timing and appropriateness of treatment with antibiotics is discussed here.

Keywords Catheters • Long term • Colonization

What Are the Risk Factors for Development of a Catheter-Associated UTI?

The duration of catheterization is the single most important risk factor. Each day that a urinary catheter is in situ, it is associated with a 5 % increase in bacteriuria [1]. Therefore, by the end of the third week, one can assume that all patients with urinary catheters will have a bacteriuria.

Other risk factors include diabetes, renal impairment, poor catheter insertion technique, poor catheter care, and colonization of the drainage bag, and female patients are at higher risk.

U.B. Mufti, MBBSc, MRCS
Department of Urology and Molecular Oncology,
Imperial Healthcare NHS Trust, Charing Cross Hospital, London, UK

R. Dasgupta, MBBChir, MA, MD, FRCS (Urol) (✉)
Department of Urology, Imperial College Healthcare NHS Trust,
St Mary's Hospital, Praed Street, London W2 1NY, UK
e-mail: ranandg@yahoo.co.uk

A. Rané, R. Dasgupta (eds.), *Urinary Tract Infection*,
DOI 10.1007/978-1-4471-4709-1_6, © Springer-Verlag London 2013

What Enables Bacteria to Enter the Catheter?

Bacteria can ascend the catheter by two mechanisms, either intraluminal or extraluminal. Intraluminal ascent of bacteria typically occurs via taps on drainage bags and during disconnection of the catheter from the bag. Extraluminal ascent occurs via biofilm formation between the catheter and the urethral mucosa. Biofilm is extremely difficult to remove, as it is well protected from mechanical flushing, host defenses, and antibiotics. Most catheter-associated UTIs derive from the colonic flora of the patient, which ascends into the bladder via the extraluminal route.

What Problems Do Patients with Long-Term Catheters Have?

Long-term catheters are likely to be colonized by bacteria, but are generally asymptomatic, and do not often account for febrile episodes in patients. However, some studies do show a relationship between long-term, catheter-associated UTI and mortality [2]. It is important to note that long-term catheters can lead to infections such as prostatitis, epididymitis, and scrotal abscess.

Noninfective complications include encrustations and catheter blockages, which in turn may become infected. Infection stones in the bladder are commonly associated with organisms such as *Klebsiella* or *Proteus* spp., as well as the commoner bacteria such as *E. coli*; the matrix that is generated by these organisms then develop into stone. Removal of a catheter with a bladder stone formed around its tip may require surgery, sometimes in the form of open surgery of the bladder. Whereas bladder stones can be treated endoscopically in most cases (i.e., transurethral surgery to perform a "cystolitholopaxy"), in a similar fashion to endoscopic prostate surgery, removal of a blocked urethral catheter would rely on a suprapubic approach (and whichever energy source is available, such as laser or pneumatic lithotripsy, to break the stone).

What Can Be Done to Reduce the Risk of Catheter-Associated UTI?

Technique: Insertion of the catheter should be done under aseptic conditions and with plenty of urethral lubricating local anesthetic.

Antibiotics: Some centers recommend use of a prophylactic dose of antibiotic prior to catheter insertion, particularly in certain high-risk patients (e.g., neuropaths, immunocompromised). However, any such protocol should be implemented in conjunction with the local microbiology department, with knowledge of microbiological flora patterns, antibiotic resistance trends, and the particular local infection rates. Choice of antibiotic will also differ, with some units recommending a single parenteral dose of an agent such as an aminoglycoside, others a single oral dose of a quinolone, or others suggesting a short course of a broad-spectrum agent immediately before and after catheter insertion.

Drainage: Patients may wish to use flip-flow valves rather than drainage bags, though there is no evidence to suggest these are more prone to infection.

Change catheter: There is much debate as to how often long-term urethral catheters require changing, but no consensus. There is a lot of current research into the effectiveness of certain catheter coatings in preventing infection; silver oxide and antibiotic-impregnated catheters are being studied. The benefit of antibiotic-impregnated catheters seems to be apparent if the catheter is in place for <1 week according to one meta-analysis (but not if in situ for >1 week) [3].

Position of catheter: there is no clearly proven benefit of suprapubic catheter as opposed to urethral catheter in terms of UTI rates, though there are clear advantages in terms of ease of changing, avoiding perineal complications, and the suprapubic route is favored for those who cannot perform self-catheterization and who need long-term urinary drainage.

What Are the Guidelines for the Treatment of Asymptomatic Bacteriuria?

There is no evidence to support the routine antibiotic treatment of asymptomatic bacteriuria. Generally, the bacteriuria will not be eradicated or will return rapidly [4]. Bacteria that re-accumulate have a higher incidence of resistance to the antibiotic used. For example, a study in which cephalexin was used showed reinfecting organisms in the control group remained susceptible to cephalexin, compared with only 36 % in the cephalexin treatment group [5].

There are some circumstances in which treatment may be beneficial. The European and Asian guidelines on Management of Catheter-associated Urinary Tract Infections recommend treatment in the following circumstances:

1. In patients undergoing urological surgery
2. To prevent nosocomial infection in the presence of a known virulent pathogen
3. Immunosuppressed patients or those at high risk of complications
4. Infection caused by strains causing a high incidence of bacteremia [4]

Treatment of Symptomatic UTI in a Catheterized Patient

Treatment is recommended in symptomatic infection. The most common manifestation is fever, but other sources must be considered. A positive urine culture cannot be regarded as diagnostic, as all patients with a long-term catheter will have bacteriuria. If safe to do so, the catheter should be replaced and antibiotic treatment started according to local protocol. Empirical antibiotic treatment should be started and subsequently modified according to urine culture results. There is no consensus on the recommended length of treatment, but antibiotics should be given for at least 5 days and up to 3 weeks, depending upon the organism and clinical state of the patient [4].

Should the Bladder Be Checked If There Is a Long-Term Catheter in Place?

There is thought to be a risk of squamous cell carcinoma where there is long-term exposure to catheters (whether indwelling or self-catheterization) or chronic infection. Endoscopic surveillance by flexible cystoscopy is therefore performed in some centers from 10 years onward, in patients with long-term drainage systems. The European Urology Association guidelines advocate annual surveillance from 10 years on, though the evidence for this is also debatable.

Is a Urinary Catheter Better Than a Condom-Based Catheter with Respect to UTIs?

The use of an indwelling catheter is for slightly different indications to a condom-based (convene) drainage system. The latter is generally to help with incontinent patients, who have urgency incontinence or who cannot reach the toilet in time before urinary leakage occurs. The indwelling catheter is used generally to allow continuous drainage (e.g., if voiding problems, in which the bladder cannot drain without assistance) and inherently carries higher risk of infection due to its invasive nature.

How Best to Drain an Infected Bladder?

A non-drained bladder becomes a reservoir for infection and culminates in "pyocystis" (a pus-filled bladder). This should be removed (cystectomy) with urinary diversion of the upper tracts (e.g., by a urinary conduit into a stoma), rather than long-term drainage by catheter. Often such patients may be deemed unfit to tolerate a cystectomy procedure and therefore may simply undergo urinary diversion. However, with time there is increased risk of overwhelming sepsis associated with leaving the infected bladder in situ, and, thus, removal of the bladder is preferable to leaving with a long-term catheter.

What Is the Best Type of Self-Catheter?

There are a number of lubricated catheters that can be used for self-catheterization, and the local facilities and resources may help determine which type is favored. There are studies comparing certain attributes of different catheters, but the general principles and technique outweigh any great differences in UTI rates.

References

1. Saint S, Meddings JA, Calfee D, Kowalski CP, Krein SL. Catheter-associated urinary tract infection and the Medicare rule changes. Ann Intern Med. 2009;150(12):877–84.
2. Emori TG, Banerjee SN, Culver DH, Gaynes RP, Horan TC, Edwards JR, Jarvis WR, Tolson JS, Henderson TS, Martone WJ, et al. Nosocomial infections in elderly patients in the United States, 1986-1990. National Nosocomial Infections Surveillance System. Am J Med. 1991;91(3B):289S–93.
3. Schumm K, Lam TB. Types of urethral catheters for the management of short-term voiding problems in hospitalized adults: a short version Cochrane review. Neurourol Urodyn. 2008;27(8):738–46.
4. Tenke P, Kovacs B, Bjerklund Johansen TE, Matsumoto T, Tambyah PA, Naber KG. European and Asian guidelines on management and prevention of catheter-associated urinary tract infections. Int J Antimicrob Agents. 2008;31 Suppl 1:S68–78.
5. Warren JW, Anthony WC, Hoopes JM, Muncie Jr HL. Cephalexin for susceptible bacteriuria in afebrile, long-term catheterized patients. JAMA. 1982;248(4):454–8.

Chapter 7
Complementary Therapy Strategies: Myths, Facts, and Lifestyle

Henry A. Lee and Dominic King

Abstract The objective of this chapter is to consider widely held popular beliefs surrounding UTIs and to see whether they stand up when scrutinized by medical research.

A great deal has been written on the subject of cranberry juice and its role in the treatment and prevention of UTIs. Cranberry juice can help prevent recurrent UTIs in women, but there is no evidence that it is effective in treating UTIs. Cranberry products work by inhibiting pathogenic adherence to the uroepithelium and probably not through acidification of the urine as was previously thought. Uva ursi (bearberry) can be used to treat UTIs affecting the lower tract, but should not be used for long-term prophylaxis as prolonged exposure to metabolites may be carcinogenic.

There is some weak evidence to suggest that probiotics and some vitamins (e.g., vitamin C) can help prevent UTIs. In addition to this, there is an association between frequency of sexual intercourse and UTIs, but not between number of partners and UTIs. Bubble bath probably does not increase the risk of UTIs, whereas condom use and contraceptive diaphragm use are associated with higher rates of UTI, although this should not discourage the use of safe sex.

Keywords Urinary tract infection • Complementary therapy • Cranberry juice • Probiotics • Vitamins • Sexual intercourse • Contraception

H.A. Lee, BSc, MBBCh, MRCS (Eng) (✉) •
D. King, BSc, MBChB, MEd, MRCS
Division of Surgery, Department of Surgery and Cancer,
Imperial College London, London, UK
e-mail: h.lee@imperial.ac.uk

A. Rané, R. Dasgupta (eds.), *Urinary Tract Infection,*
DOI 10.1007/978-1-4471-4709-1_7, © Springer-Verlag London 2013

What Complementary Therapies Can Be Used in the Management of UTIs?

In the last decade, there has been widespread and increasing interest from Western populations in complementary therapies (also known as alternative therapy or medicine, natural remedies or therapy, or traditional therapy). Such therapies are used for many conditions, but there is a more widespread acceptance of their use for UTIs. The most popular, and most formally investigated, is cranberry juice or cranberry products [1]. Numerous other botanicals, such as berberine [2], blueberry [3], and uva ursi (bearberry) [4], have also been investigated, as have naturally occurring nutrients, such as vitamin C [5] and D–mannose [6], as well as probiotics [7, 8]. Nearly all complementary therapies used in relation to UTIs are for infections of the lower rather than upper urinary tract.

Can Cranberry Juice or Products Be Used to Treat UTIs?

Popular urban myths and "old wives" tales abound regarding the use of cranberry juice in the treatment of UTIs. A number of recent and methodologically robust systematic reviews have concluded that there is no evidence to suggest that cranberry juice, or cranberry products, are effective at treating UTIs [9–11].

Cranberry bush with fruit partially submerged

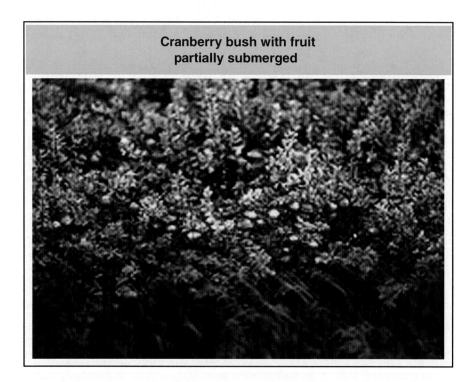

Cranberry bush with fruit partially submerged

Can Cranberry Juice or Products Be Used to Prevent UTIs?

A Cochrane review and meta-analysis of the use of cranberry products in the prevention of UTIs concluded that over a 12-month period, daily use significantly reduced the incidence of UTIs [9]. The authors commented that the evidence was strongest for women with recurrent UTIs. There is mixed evidence to support the use of cranberry products in elderly populations [12]. There is no evidence to suggest that cranberry products are of benefit for preventing symptomatic UTIs in individuals with long-term urinary catheters [13].

There are many different cranberry product formulations and the recommended dose varies, depending upon the brand and concentration. The usual dose for UTI prevention is 250–500 ml daily and unsweetened juice is preferable [14]. Capsules that contain concentrated cranberry juice are a popular alternative and are usually taken two to three times a day for prevention [14]. It should be noted that although the popular conception of a glass of cranberry juice a day to prevent UTIs is an easy form of therapy to follow, the evidence would suggest otherwise. Compliance rates of less than 80 % are not uncommon, and in one study 63 % of participants dropped out [15], suggesting that cranberry products may not be acceptable for long-term use.

How Do Cranberry Products Prevent UTIs?

Cranberries (*Vaccinium macrocarpon*) have been used to treat and prevent UTIs for centuries as part of different folk remedies. There are two main mechanisms through which cranberry products are thought to prevent UTIs, acidification of urine and inhibition of bacterial adherence to the urothelium.

The acidification theory is a straightforward one and suggests that the quinic acid in cranberry juice causes large amounts of hippuric acid to be secreted in the urine [16]. The lowered pH of the urine creates an inhospitable environment for uropathogens. Doubt has been cast over this theory, however [1], as only short-lived reductions in urinary pH have been seen in more recent studies where participants have ingested usual amounts of cranberry products [17, 18]. A different explanation is that the ingestion of these products prevents pathogenic bacteria from adhering to the lining of the urinary tract. Cranberry products have been shown to prevent pathogenic adherence to the urothelium through interfering with fimbrial binding to epithelial cells [19]. Several different fruit juices (including guava, mango, grapefruit, and blueberry) have been shown to inhibit bacterial adherence related to type 1 fimbrial expression (mannose sensitive), whereas only cranberry juice and blueberry juice have been shown to reduce adherence related to type P fimbrial expression [3, 20].

Do Cranberry Products Interact with Other Medications?

Cranberry products are generally very safe. The main issue surrounding their use has been a possible interaction with warfarin. Based on 12 reports of possible interactions with warfarin [21], the British Committee on Safety of Medicines and the Medicines and Healthcare Products Regulatory Agency issued advice that patients taking cranberry juice with warfarin should have their international normalized ratio (INR) monitored closely [22]. A subsequent systematic review has, however, shown no available data to support cranberry juice as the agent responsible for the INR elevations [23].

What Other Botanicals Can Help Prevent UTIs?

Blueberries (*Vaccinium myrtillus*), also known as bilberries, are thought to help prevent UTIs through a similar mechanism as cranberries [3], although blueberry juice is less acidic. There is certainly less evidence from clinical practice to support blueberry use, although this may, in part at least, be due to the fact that cranberry juice has been more widely available for a longer period than blueberry juice. Given that blueberries have gained "superfood" status in the popular press [24, 25], it is likely that more work will be forthcoming in this area in the near future. Guidelines on the effective dose or volume of blueberry product to prevent UTIs are difficult to obtain and vary, depending upon the brand and concentration purchased.

Blueberry (Wikipedia)

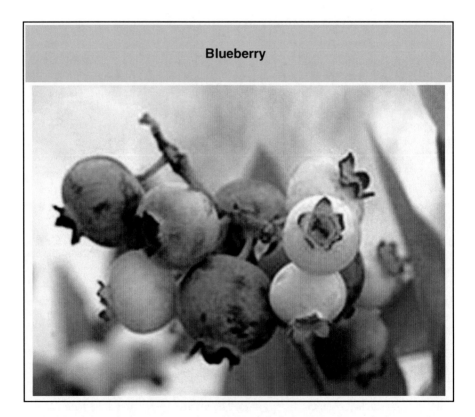

Berberine is a plant isoquinoline alkaloid that is yellow in color and bitter to the taste. It has been used in Ayurvedic and Chinese medicine for many centuries [26] and can be found in many plants, e.g., oregon grape (*Mahonia aquifolium*), goldthread (*Coptis chinensis*), and **goldenseal** (*Hydrastis canadensis*) [27]. It has principally been used for treatment of gastrointestinal infections such as *Giardia lamblia* and *E. coli*, although its use in relation to UTIs has been reported [27]. Its mechanism of action is thought to be due to direct bacteriostatic action through inhibiting cell division [28] and prevention of bacterial adhesion [29]. Berberine, or remedies containing this supplement, should not be taken during pregnancy due to the risk of inducing uterine contractions.

Goldenseal (Wikipedia)

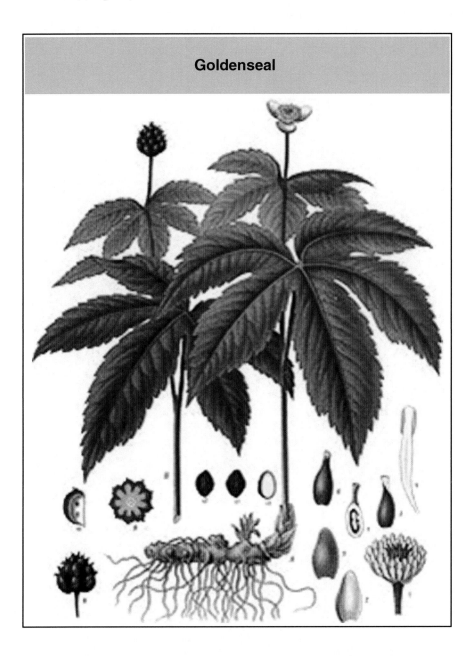

Uva ursi (*Arctostaphylos uva ursi*), also known as **bearberry**, is a shrub native to mountainous regions of North America. The leaves of the shrub contain the glycoside arbutoside, which, when ingested, is absorbed as hydroquinone and, after hepatic glucuronidation, is renally excreted [4]. The hydroquinone is spontaneously released from hydroquinone glucuronide as long as the urine is sufficiently alkali (pH > 7) and has direct antibacterial effects. Unlike cranberry products, uva ursi is used for the treatment and not prevention of UTIs and has federal licensing for treatment of UTIs in Germany [14]. It should not be taken for long-term prophylaxis, however, as there is some concern that prolonged use may be carcinogenic. The recommended dose in Germany is 3 g leaf extracted in 150 ml water by either hot or cold infusion up to four times daily, providing 400–840 mg arbutoside [14].

Bearberry (Wikipedia)

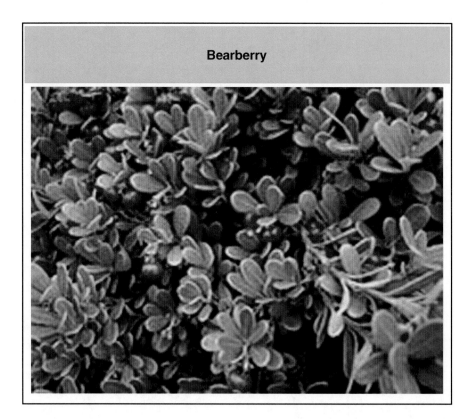

Bearberry

Juniper (*Juniperus communis*) is a tree that is found predominantly in temperate European regions and is another botanical with antimicrobial activity that has been used to treat UTIs [14]. The use of juniper tea for UTIs is a common folk remedy across Europe, and its activity is believed to be through the action of antimicrobial terpenoids that may have additional diuretic activity.

Cones and leaves from the juniper tree (Wikipedia)

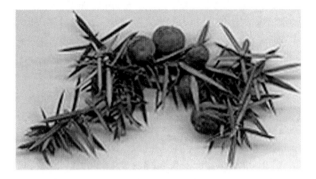

Additional botanicals that have also been used in the treatment of UTIs include buchu (*Barosma betulina*), marshmallow root (*Althea officinalis*), horsetail (*Equisetum arvense*), dandelion leaf (*Taraxacum officinale*), and corn silk (Zea mays). These complementary therapies may be as efficacious as those named above, but have not yet been as extensively investigated.

How Effective Are Probiotics at Treating and Preventing UTIs?

Probiotics are another complementary therapy that has gained popularity in recent years, with supermarkets and health-food stores carrying an increasing range of such products. Probiotics are described by the WHO as "live microorganisms, which when administered in adequate amounts confer a health benefit to the host" [30].

Probiotics famously owe their origins to an observation made by Russian Nobel Laureate Ilya Mechnikov, who attributed the long life and good health of Bulgarian peasants to their consumption of large quantities of yogurt that contained lactic acid bacteria [31].

Compared to their application in gastrointestinal conditions, the use of probiotics in the treatment of UTIs has been the focus of much less medical research [7, 8], although there have been several trials investigating their use in preventing recurrent UTIs [32–35]. The results of these, however, have not consistently upheld the use of probiotics, and in fact, only one trial reported a significant reduction in recurrent episodes [32]. These studies have almost exclusively been undertaken in young women with recurrent UTIs, and there is little evidence to demonstrate effectiveness in other groups.

Can Vitamins Be Used to Treat UTIs?

There is some evidence to support the use of vitamins, but no body of work proves that they can replace more conventional therapies in treating infections. Vitamin C, for example, is a complementary therapy that is widely believed to be beneficial in treating UTIs [36], yet despite its popularity on the high street for this purpose, the evidence to support a direct effect of vitamin C in treating UTIs is not overwhelming. Vitamin C has been shown in small studies to be useful in helping to prevent urinary tract infections in pregnant women [5] and has been shown to help protect against UTI in a case-controlled study of college-aged women [37]. Vitamin A has also received some attention in respect to the prevention of UTIs, although mainly in pediatric populations. There is limited evidence to support its use in conjunction with initial antimicrobial therapy [38], although results are far from conclusive [39].

Potassium and sodium citrate salts have been used in the alkalinizing of urine and are a commonly used complementary therapy that has been widely adopted by the medical community. Their effect is brought through raising the pH of the urine and, in doing so, inhibiting microbial pathogenesis. They are particularly efficacious in treating symptomatic dysuria [40] and help potentiate the effects of certain botanicals such as uva ursi. D–Mannose is another nutrient that is a popular complementary therapy for treating UTIs [27, 41]. Pathogenic *E. coli* bind to the urinary tract via a specific mannose-sensitive receptor mechanism [42, 43], and by increasing urinary mannose through dietary supplementation, bacterial adherence and subsequent pathogenesis can be reduced. There is, however, no clinical trial data demonstrating the efficacy or otherwise of D–mannose in humans.

Can Acupuncture Help Prevent UTIs?

Acupuncture is suggested as an effective means of preventing UTIs by alternative therapy stores and in the self-help literature. Unfortunately, this seems to amount to little more than unproven enthusiasm. Other than numerous individual testimonials, a literature search found only one trial into acupuncture to prevent UTIs [44], and this followed on from work by the same authors [45]. This study showed that participants in the acupuncture group developed fewer UTIs than controls, but has been criticized in terms of study design and for the conclusions made on the basis of the results [46].

Acupuncture needles being inserted into a patient's skin (Wikipedia)

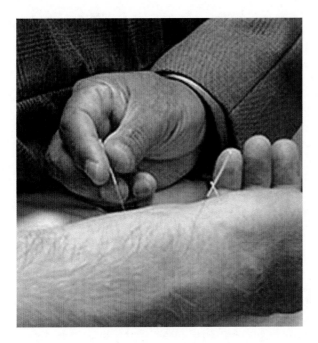

Does Having Sex Cause UTIs?

The link between heterosexual vaginal intercourse and UTIs is a popular association held by the general public and has given rise to the term "honeymoon cystitis" or "honeymoon bladder" [47]. The link between primary UTI and intercourse was suggested in a study that demonstrated that young nuns have a lower level of bacteriuria than other populations [48] and has been subsequently substantiated by cross-sectional case-control studies and prospective population-based cohort studies [49–52].

For women who suffer from recurrent UTIs, sexual intercourse has also been shown to be a strong predictor of developing a symptomatic infection [53], and other works on college populations have shown that sexual intercourse increased the risk of recurrent UTI in women, with both a different and the same uropathogen as the first UTI [54].

Is There a Link Between Number of Sexual Partners and UTIs?

Generally speaking, UTIs are not regarded as sexually transmitted infections, and as such there is no link between the number of sexual partners and UTIs [37, 51, 55]. There is, however, an association between the *frequency* of intercourse and UTIs [52]. Unmarried young women having vaginal intercourse more than seven times per week have been shown to have a nine times increased risk of UTI, compared to those who did not have sexual intercourse during this period, with investigators demonstrating a dose-response relation between recent sexual intercourse and the risk of UTI [49].

Does Drinking Lots of Water Help Treat a UTI?

The belief that "flushing out" infections is one that is firmly fixed in the consciousness of the general public and of healthcare professionals alike. The evidence to support this, however, is far from clear and is contradictory to a degree [56, 57]. Studies in the 1960s based on reproductive rates of bacterial pathogens, prior to knowledge that bacteria adherence was integral to virulence, demonstrated that flow alone was not sufficient to flush out bacteria when voided volumes were small [58].

It is certainly the case that individuals with UTI should avoid dehydration to ensure optimal immune function and that any concomitant antimicrobial treatment is effective. There is evidence that many women with recurrent UTIs are helped by a fluid intake or more than 2 l/day [59]. Perhaps the most well-balanced advice is from Kunin, who suggests that "instruction to patients to drink ample fluids and void frequently appears to be justifiable, except when the patient is being treated for infection with agents that need to be concentrated in the urine" [60].

Can Drinking Carbonated or Caffeinated Drinks Cause UTIs?

Internet forums for UTIs and health self-help websites repeatedly advocate avoiding carbonated and caffeinated drinks (such as cola, tea, and coffee), but to say that they cause UTIs is untrue. These beverages may, however, mimic or exacerbate symptoms of a UTI and have been associated with increased rates of UTIs in some populations.

Caffeine is believed to increase detrusor pressure [61] and also acts as a mild diuretic, so it may exacerbate the lower urinary tract symptoms associated with a

UTI. Regular consumption of cola drinks and tea has been shown in some studies to be strongly associated with UTIs, as have coffee and other carbonated drinks to a lesser extent [36], although another work has not demonstrated these links [50]. Preliminary results from a more recent study suggest that tea, coffee, and cola are all strongly associated with developing UTIs [62].

Are There Any Other Popular Misconceptions About Lifestyle Factors and UTIs?

One popular myth states that the wearing of tight-fitting clothes can predispose to UTIs. Not much formal work has been done into this area, but one study of college-aged women showed that wearing tight jeans, as compared to loose/very loose jeans, was strongly associated with first UTI, and moderately associated with second UTI [36]. Wearing cotton underwear is commonly regarded as helpful in preventing UTI, although there is no evidence to support this widely held belief, and one study showed an association between first UTI and wearing cotton underwear [36]. There was a slight association between bubble baths and UTIs in one study, but no other evidence to convincingly support or refute the well-known claim that bubble baths predispose to UTIs. However, there is good evidence that contraceptive diaphragms are associated with UTIs [50, 63], as is condom use [52, 64].

Key Points
- Cranberry juice can help prevent recurrent UTIs in women, but there is no evidence that it is effective in treating UTIs.
- Cranberry products work by inhibiting pathogenic adherence to the uroepithelium and probably not through acidification of the urine as was previously thought.
- Uva ursi can be used to treat UTIs affecting the lower tract, but should not be used for long-term prophylaxis as prolonged exposure to metabolites may be carcinogenic.
- There is some weak evidence to suggest that probiotics and some vitamins can help prevent UTIs.
- There is an association between frequency of sexual intercourse and UTIs, but not between number of partners and UTIs.
- Bubble baths probably do not increase the risk of UTIs, whereas condom use and contraceptive diaphragm use are associated with higher rates of UTI.

References

1. Jepson RG, Craig JC. Cranberries for preventing urinary tract infections. Cochrane Database Syst Rev 2008;(1):CD001321.
2. Cernakova M, Kostalova D. Antimicrobial activity of berberine – a constituent of Mahonia aquifolium. Folia Microbiol (Praha). 2002;47(4):375–8.
3. Ofek I, Goldhar J, Zafriri D, Lis H, Adar R, Sharon N. Anti-Escherichia coli adhesion activity of cranberry and blueberry juices. N Engl J Med. 1991;324(22):1599.
4. Schindler G, Patzak U, Brinkhaus B, von Niecieck A, Wittig J, Krahmer N, Glockl I, Veit M. Urinary excretion and metabolism of arbutin after oral administration of Arctostaphylos uvae ursi extract as film-coated tablets and aqueous solution in healthy humans. J Clin Pharmacol. 2002;42(8):920–7.
5. Ochoa-Brust GJ, Fernandez AR, Villanueva-Ruiz GJ, Velasco R, Trujillo-Hernandez B, Vasquez C. Daily intake of 100 mg ascorbic acid as urinary tract infection prophylactic agent during pregnancy. Acta Obstet Gynecol Scand. 2007;86(7):783–7.
6. Schaeffer AJ, Chmiel JS, Duncan JL, Falkowski WS. Mannose-sensitive adherence of Escherichia coli to epithelial cells from women with recurrent urinary tract infections. J Urol. 1984;131(5):906–10.
7. Borchert D, Sheridan L, Papatsoris A, Faruquz Z, Barua JM, Junaid I, Pati Y, Chinegwundoh F, Buchholz N. Prevention and treatment of urinary tract infection with probiotics: review and research perspective. Indian J Urol. 2008;24(2):139–44.
8. de Vrese M. Health benefits of probiotics and prebiotics in women. Menopause Int. 2009;15(1):35–40.
9. Jepson RG, Mihaljevic L, Craig J. Cranberries for treating urinary tract infections. Cochrane Database Syst Rev 2000;(2):CD001322.
10. Griffiths P. The role of cranberry juice in the treatment of urinary tract infections. Br J Community Nurs. 2003;8(12):557–61.
11. Santillo VM, Lowe FC. Cranberry juice for the prevention and treatment of urinary tract infections. Drugs Today (Barc). 2007;43(1):47–54.
12. Sumukadas D, Davey P, McMurdo ME. Recurrent urinary tract infections in older people: the role of cranberry products. Age Ageing. 2009;38(3):255–7.
13. Jepson RG, Mihaljevic L, Craig J. Cranberries for preventing urinary tract infections. Cochrane Database Syst Rev 2004;(2):CD001321.
14. Yarnell E. Botanical medicines for the urinary tract. World J Urol. 2002;20(5):285–93.
15. Foda MM, Middlebrook PF, Gatfield CT, Potvin G, Wells G, Schillinger JF. Efficacy of cranberry in prevention of urinary tract infection in a susceptible pediatric population. Can J Urol. 1995;2(1):98–102.
16. Fellers CR. Nutritive value of cranberries. Am J Public Health Nations Health. 1933;23(1):13–8.
17. McLeod DC, Nahata MC. Methenamine therapy and urine acidification with ascorbic acid and cranberry juice. Am J Hosp Pharm. 1978;35(6):654.
18. Kahn HD, Panariello VA, Saeli J, Sampson JR, Schwartz E. Effect of cranberry juice on urine. J Am Diet Assoc. 1967;51(3):251–4.
19. Zafriri D, Ofek I, Adar R, Pocino M, Sharon N. Inhibitory activity of cranberry juice on adherence of type 1 and type P fimbriated Escherichia coli to eucaryotic cells. Antimicrob Agents Chemother. 1989;33(1):92–8.
20. Ofek I, Goldhar J, Sharon N. Anti-Escherichia coli adhesin activity of cranberry and blueberry juices. Adv Exp Med Biol. 1996;408:179–83.
21. Sylvan L, Justice NP. Possible interaction between warfarin and cranberry juice. Am Fam Physician. 2005;72(6):1000; author reply 1000.
22. Committee on Safety of Medicines MaHPRA. Interaction between warfarin and cranberry juice: new advice. Curr Probl Pharmacovigil. 2004;30:10.
23. Pham DQ, Pham AQ. Interaction potential between cranberry juice and warfarin. Am J Health Syst Pharm. 2007;64(5):490–4.

24. Kirby T. Blueberries: shoppers lap up UK's new superfood. The Independent. Tuesday, 17 May 2005.
25. Pratt S, Matthews K. SuperFoods Rx: fourteen foods that will change your life. New York: Harper; 2006.
26. Kaneda Y, Torii M, Tanaka T, Aikawa M. In vitro effects of berberine sulphate on the growth and structure of Entamoeba histolytica, Giardia lamblia and Trichomonas vaginalis. Ann Trop Med Parasitol. 1991;85(4):417–25.
27. Head KA. Natural approaches to prevention and treatment of infections of the lower urinary tract. Altern Med Rev. 2008;13(3):227–44.
28. Domadia PN, Bhunia A, Sivaraman J, Swarup S, Dasgupta D. Berberine targets assembly of Escherichia coli cell division protein FtsZ. Biochemistry. 2008;47(10):3225–34.
29. Sun D, Abraham SN, Beachey EH. Influence of berberine sulfate on synthesis and expression of Pap fimbrial adhesin in uropathogenic Escherichia coli. Antimicrob Agents Chemother. 1988;32(8):1274–7.
30. FAO/WHO. Health and nutritional properties of probiotics in food including powder milk with live lactic acid bacteria. Report of a joint FAO/WHO expert consultation on evaluation of health and nutritional properties of probiotics in food including powder milk with live lactic acid bacteria. 2001.
31. Parkes GC. An overview of probiotics and prebiotics. Nurs Stand. 2007;21(20):43–7.
32. Reid G, Bruce AW, Taylor M. Influence of three-day antimicrobial therapy and lactobacillus vaginal suppositories on recurrence of urinary tract infections. Clin Ther. 1992;14(1):11–6.
33. Baerheim A, Larsen E, Digranes A. Vaginal application of lactobacilli in the prophylaxis of recurrent lower urinary tract infection in women. Scand J Prim Health Care. 1994;12(4):239–43.
34. Reid G, Bruce A, Taylor M. Instillation of Lactobacillus and stimulation of indigenous organisms to prevent recurrence of urinary tract infections. Microecol Ther. 1995;23:32–45.
35. Kontiokari T, Sundqvist K, Nuutinen M, Pokka T, Koskela M, Uhari M. Randomised trial of cranberry-lingonberry juice and Lactobacillus GG drink for the prevention of urinary tract infections in women. BMJ. 2001;322(7302):1571.
36. Foxman B, Frerichs RR. Epidemiology of urinary tract infection: II. Diet, clothing, and urination habits. Am J Public Health. 1985;75(11):1314–7.
37. Foxman B, Chi JW. Health behavior and urinary tract infection in college-aged women. J Clin Epidemiol. 1990;43(4):329–37.
38. Yilmaz A, Bahat E, Yilmaz GG, Hasanoglu A, Akman S, Guven AG. Adjuvant effect of vitamin A on recurrent lower urinary tract infections. Pediatr Int. 2007;49(3):310–3.
39. Williams G, Craig JC. Prevention of recurrent urinary tract infection in children. Curr Opin Infect Dis. 2009;22(1):72–6.
40. Spooner JB. Alkalinisation in the management of cystitis. J Int Med Res. 1984;12(1):30–4.
41. d-Mannose.co.uk. http://www.d-mannose.co.uk/. Last Accessed 27 Sept 2009.
42. Martinez JJ, Mulvey MA, Schilling JD, Pinkner JS, Hultgren SJ. Type 1 pilus-mediated bacterial invasion of bladder epithelial cells. EMBO J. 2000;19(12):2803–12.
43. Hung CS, Bouckaert J, Hung D, Pinkner J, Widberg C, DeFusco A, Auguste CG, Strouse R, Langermann S, Waksman G, Hultgren SJ. Structural basis of tropism of Escherichia coli to the bladder during urinary tract infection. Mol Microbiol. 2002;44(4):903–15.
44. Alraek T, Soedal LI, Fagerheim SU, Digranes A, Baerheim A. Acupuncture treatment in the prevention of uncomplicated recurrent lower urinary tract infections in adult women. Am J Public Health. 2002;92(10):1609–11.
45. Aune A, Alraek T, LiHua H, Baerheim A. Acupuncture in the prophylaxis of recurrent lower urinary tract infection in adult women. Scand J Prim Health Care. 1998;16(1):37–9.
46. Katz AR. Urinary tract infections and acupuncture. Am J Public Health. 2003;93(5):702; author reply 702–3.
47. Ronald A. Sex and urinary tract infections. N Engl J Med. 1996;335(7):511–2.
48. Kunin CM, McCormack RC. An epidemiologic study of bacteriuria and blood pressure among nuns and working women. N Engl J Med. 1968;278(12):635–42.

49. Hooton TM, Scholes D, Hughes JP, Winter C, Roberts PL, Stapleton AE, Stergachis A, Stamm WE. A prospective study of risk factors for symptomatic urinary tract infection in young women. N Engl J Med. 1996;335(7):468–74.
50. Remis RS, Gurwith MJ, Gurwith D, Hargrett-Bean NT, Layde PM. Risk factors for urinary tract infection. Am J Epidemiol. 1987;126(4):685–94.
51. Strom BL, Collins M, West SL, Kreisberg J, Weller S. Sexual activity, contraceptive use, and other risk factors for symptomatic and symptomatic bacteriuria. A case-control study. Ann Intern Med. 1987;107(6):816–23.
52. Foxman B, Geiger AM, Palin K, Gillespie B, Koopman JS. First-time urinary tract infection and sexual behavior. Epidemiology. 1995;6(2):162–8.
53. Czaja CA, Stamm WE, Stapleton AE, Roberts PL, Hawn TR, Scholes D, Samadpour M, Hultgren SJ, Hooton TM. Prospective cohort study of microbial and inflammatory events immediately preceding Escherichia coli recurrent urinary tract infection in women. J Infect Dis. 2009;200(4):528–36.
54. Foxman B, Gillespie B, Koopman J, Zhang L, Palin K, Tallman P, Marsh JV, Spear S, Sobel JD, Marty MJ, Marrs CF. Risk factors for second urinary tract infection among college women. Am J Epidemiol. 2000;151(12):1194–205.
55. Kelsey MC, Mead MG, Gruneberg RN, Oriel JD. Relationship between sexual intercourse and urinary-tract infection in women attending a clinic for sexually transmitted diseases. J Med Microbiol. 1979;12(4):511–2.
56. Reid G. Potential preventive strategies and therapies in urinary tract infection. World J Urol. 1999;17(6):359–63.
57. Beetz R. Mild dehydration: a risk factor of urinary tract infection? Eur J Clin Nutr. 2003;57 Suppl 2:S52–8.
58. Boen JR, Sylwester DL. The mathematical relationship among urinary frequency, residual urine, and bacterial growth in bladder infections. Invest Urol. 1965;2:468–73.
59. Bailey RR. Management of uncomplicated urinary tract infections. Int J Antimicrob Agents. 1994;4(2):95–100.
60. Kunin CM. Detection, prevention and management of urinary tract infections. Philadelphia: Lea & Febiger; 1987.
61. Creighton SM, Stanton SL. Caffeine: does it affect your bladder? Br J Urol. 1990;66(6): 613–4.
62. Vincent C. Symptoms and risk factors associated with a first UTI in college-aged women: a prospective cohort study. AUA. 2009;2009:Abstract 396.
63. Foxman B, Frerichs RR. Epidemiology of urinary tract infection: I. Diaphragm use and sexual intercourse. Am J Public Health. 1985;75(11):1308–13.
64. Foxman B, Marsh J, Gillespie B, Rubin N, Koopman JS, Spear S. Condom use and first-time urinary tract infection. Epidemiology. 1997;8(6):637–41.

Chapter 8
A Look to the Future

Ranan Dasgupta

Abstract The development of guidelines for management of urinary tract infections has helped toward some standardization in this diverse field, though it is becoming increasingly apparent how limited our antibiotic armamentarium is becoming, through the development of resistant bacteria. Clearly new treatment strategies are needed (e.g., vaccination), and we await clinical trials to test such novel therapies which are much needed.

Keywords UTI • Guidelines • Vaccinations • Antimicrobial

Bacteria have existed for several million years, and therefore the discovery of penicillin in the past century would seem to be a footnote in history, and the development of subsequent antibiotic resistance appears like a postscript. The widespread application of antibiotics incorporates prophylactic and therapeutic regimes to manage urinary tract infections, both community-acquired and nosocomial in origin.

Guidelines are developed by specialist organizations which could perhaps address the different challenges for UTIs in the community and in the hospital setting, and while local variations will always exist, a global perspective (e.g., through international databases, such as that exemplified by the Working Group for UTI in the European Association of Urology) would be particularly useful. Antibiotic prophylaxis before surgery has been adopted as a universally accepted principle, and therefore, such knowledge would help rationalize and optimize treatment regimens.

Future research in this field may include strategies against recurrent infections (e.g., vaccines [1, 2]), minimizing antibiotic resistance (possibly as a public health intervention, in the laboratory, or likely both), identifying the genetic predisposition

R. Dasgupta, MBBChir, MA, MD, FRCS (Urol)
Department of Urology, Imperial College Healthcare NHS Trust,
St Mary's Hospital, Praed Street, London W2 1NY, UK
e-mail: ranandg@yahoo.co.uk

A. Rané, R. Dasgupta (eds.), *Urinary Tract Infection*,
DOI 10.1007/978-1-4471-4709-1_8, © Springer-Verlag London 2013

to recurrent infections, and further development of technologies to deliver antimicrobial treatments (e.g., drug-eluting stents or other devices).

In some ways, a short book such as this can answer some of the basic questions of how best to manage UTIs, but hopefully readers will also be sufficiently challenged to enquire how to improve care in certain conditions and be stimulated into perhaps even finding the solutions.

References

1. Zakri RH, Dasgupta R, Dasgupta P, Khan MS. Preventing recurrent urinary infections: role of vaccines. BJU Int. 2008;102(9):1055–6.
2. Zaffanello M, Malerba G, Cataldi L, et al. Genetic risk for recurrent UTIs in humans: a systematic review. J Biomed Biotechnol. 2010.

Index

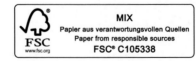

Printed by Books on Demand, Germany